The Global Burden of Disease and Risk Factors - Understanding and Management

Edited by Mukadder Mollaoğlu and Murat Can Mollaoğlu

Published in London, United Kingdom

The Global Burden of Disease and Risk Factors - Understanding and Management
http://dx.doi.org/10.5772/intechopen.111121
Edited by Mukadder Mollaoğlu and Murat Can Mollaoğlu

Contributors
Abdelilah El Abbassi, Anna Mihailova, Ayaka Sudo, Behzad Saberi, Deshi Dong, Es-Said Sabir, Fatema Akter, Hanane Moummou, Hicham Chatoui, Hiromi Hamano, Hitoshi Sohma, Hong Xiang, Imane Meftah, Iman Meftah, Jamal Karoumi, Lahoucine Bahi, Linlin Lv, Maximiliane Trapp, Michitoshi Kimura, Mihoko Ohashi, Mounia Achoch, Mounia Akhallaayoune, Mounir Tilaoui, Murat Can Mollaoğlu, Nahid Shamandi, Natalija Kakurina, Omar El Hiba, Oumnia Akhallaayoune, Rafael Suárez del Villar Carrero, Sanjeev Kumar, Weny Rinawati, Xufeng Tao, Yasuo Kokai

First published in London, United Kingdom, 2024 by IntechOpen
IntechOpen is the global imprint of INTECHOPEN LIMITED, registered in England and Wales, registration number: 11086078, 167-169 Great Portland Street, London, W1W 5PF, United Kingdom

British Library Cataloguing-in-Publication Data
A catalogue record for this book is available from the British Library

Additional hard and PDF copies can be obtained from orders@intechopen.com

The Global Burden of Disease and Risk Factors - Understanding and Management
Edited by Mukadder Mollaoğlu and Murat Can Mollaoğlu
p. cm.
Print ISBN 978-0-85466-086-5
Online ISBN 978-0-85466-085-8
eBook (PDF) ISBN 978-0-85466-087-2

Meet the editors

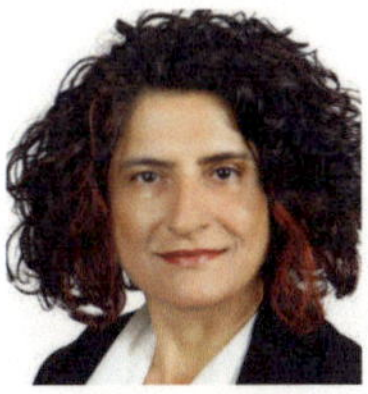

Professor Mukadder Mollaoğlu, Ph.D., is a member of the Faculty of Health Sciences, Sivas Cumhuriyet University, Turkey. Her areas of research interest include care management in chronic diseases, infectious disease management, psychosocial care, quality of life, life satisfaction, home care, caregivers' needs, development of self-care activities in chronic diseases, integrative therapy, self-sufficiency, and health ethics. Her research work has been published in many high-impact journals and has received numerous citations. Dr. Mollaoğlu is the editor and author of several books and book chapters.

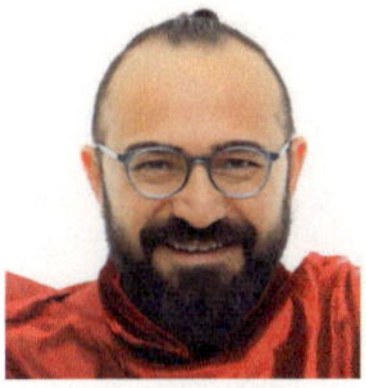

Dr. Murat Can Mollaoğlu, MD, graduated from the Faculty of Medicine, Istanbul University Cerrahpaşa, Turkey, in 2007. He became a general surgery specialist in 2016 and a subspecialist in surgical oncology in 2020. He serves patients with chronic health problems. Dr. Mollaoğlu has many journal articles and book chapters to his credit. He has also edited several books.

Contents

Preface

Understanding the global burden of lifestyle and chronic diseases is crucial for developing effective disease management strategies. This book offers insights into managing the global disease burden and discusses risk factors in three parts. Reducing the risk factors associated with these diseases is key to prevention and control.

The first part of the book examines the risk factors that contribute to the emergence of global diseases and explores different approaches to controlling these risky situations. The second part focuses on medical management, providing an understanding of global diseases and their burden. This section discusses current medical approaches to treating diseases such as Alzheimer's, neurodegenerative diseases, and traumatic brain injury. The third section includes chapters on treatment practices that support the medical approach in managing global diseases.

Each topic in this book provides important information for health professionals, students in the health field, those interested in alternative treatment methods, and especially those interested in herbal treatments. Each chapter has been prepared with great effort and aims to contribute to the literature. We express our gratitude to each author who made valuable contributions to the chapters and to IntechOpen publishing house for providing the opportunity to publish this information.

Dr. Mukadder Mollaoğlu
Professor,
Health Sciences Faculty,
Sivas Cumhuriyet University,
Sivas, Turkey

Dr. Murat Can Mollaoğlu
Assistant Professor,
İstinye University Gaziosmanpaşa Medical Park,
İstanbul, Turkey

Section 1

Management of Risk Factors in Global Diseases

Chapter 1

Global Burden of Disease Study 2019 Indicates That Smoking Gradually Becomes a Key Driver of the Burden of Pancreatic Cancer in Developing Regions

Hong Xiang, Deshi Dong, Linlin Lv and Xufeng Tao

Abstract

Pancreatic cancer (PC) remains a high mortality disease worldwide with a 5-year survival rate of less than 10%. Economic and living standard improvements in developing countries have significantly raised behavioral and metabolic risk factors of PC-related burden over the past decades. However, previous studies have not fully clarified how these risk factors contribute to PC over time. By employing the Global Burden of Disease (GBD) Study 2019, we examined PC-associated burden and its related risk factors from 1990 to 2019 in the present paper. During that time frame, the number of PC death cases significantly increased throughout the world; and developing regions have a higher trend compared to developed regions. Smoking, high fasting plasma glucose (FPG), as well as high body mass index (BMI) have become significant drivers of PC burden, which has also contributed to the rise in PC-related deaths in developing countries. Meanwhile, the rapid increase in premature deaths in developing countries should draw the public's attention. It is therefore necessary to intervene on the PC-associated risk factors to significantly reduce death cases and burden. The renewal of PC burden analysis in this paper at multiple levels in GBD database is very beneficial for each country to determine individual policies to control the increasing trend of this disease.

Keywords: pancreatic cancer, global burden of disease, risk factors, smoking, fasting plasma glucose, body mass index

1. Introduction

Pancreatic cancer (PC) is an aggressive malignancy arising from the pancreas with a poor prognosis, and its risk factors include smoking, pancreatitis, alcohol use, and a cluster of metabolic conditions such as obesity, hypertension, dyslipidemia, insulin resistance, and type 2 diabetes mellitus [1–3]. Currently, PC is the fourth leading cause of cancer-related deaths in Western societies, and it is predicted to be the second leading cause of cancer-related mortality in America in 2030 [4, 5]. Over the past decades, the rapid improvement of economy and living standards in developing countries has notably caused the promotion of metabolic risk factors (e.g., high fasting plasma glucose (FPG) and body mass index (BMI)) incidences) [6–8]. In addition, tobacco smoking is a rich and poisonous mixture that causes various diseases via multiple mechanisms, especially cancers [9, 10]. Therefore, the effects of these risk factors on PC-related death cases over time warrants investigation, and it is also gradually becoming significantly urgent for PC prevention in developing countries.

In order to prevent and manage PC, it is pivotal to obtain and analyze detailed and comparable epidemiological estimates for PC by geography, year, age, and sex, as well as the related risk factors. Global Burden of PC collaborators have shown a global overview of the epidemiology and risk factors of PC; however, PC burden has not been well understood on a worldwide scale as far as we know [11–13]. Therefore, our team summarized and further analyzed the PC-related burden between 1990 and 2019 in this paper by using the data reported in the Global Burden of Diseases, Injuries, and Risk Factors Study (GBD) 2019. Moreover, we show the results of PC-related burden in different sex and age groups and its associated burden and risk factors at global, regional, and national levels. In short, we found that PC-associated death cases significantly increased from 1990 to 2019, and high FPG and BMI as well as smoking contribute to the age-standardized death rate (ASDR) increase in low sociodemographic index (SDI) regions. Therefore, the present paper may provide critical suggestions for developing available preventive measures to decrease the PC burden around the world.

2. Methods

2.1 Data source

The 2019 GBD study provides updated and detailed burden estimates of diseases, injuries, and related risk factors at global, regional, and national levels through integrating all available data around the world. Global Health Data Exchange (GHDx) query tool is maintained by the Institute for Health Metrics and Evaluation, and it encompasses available data on over 369 human pathologies and 87 attributable risk factors, obtained from 204 different countries and territories [14, 15]. In the present paper, annual numbers and ASDRs of PC-related deaths, disability-adjusted life years (DALYs), years of life lost (YLLs), years of life lived with disability (YLDs), and incidence and prevalence rates from 1990 to 2019 were obtained via the GHDx query tool (http://ghdx.healthdata.org/gbd-results-tool).

2.2 Attributable burden estimation

Estimation methods in this paper have been described in detail in previous research [15, 16]. The natural logarithm of ASDR assumes linearity over time; therefore, $Y = \alpha + \beta X + \varepsilon$, where Y equals ln (ASDR), X equals calendar year, and ε equals error term; and ASDR's estimated annual percentage change (EAPC) was counted via the "$100 \times (\exp(\beta) - 1)$" formula [17, 18]. Having a positive EAPC indicates that the trend of the ASDR is increasing, and having a negative EAPC indicates a decreasing trend for the ASDR. Additionally, the change from 1990 to 2019 in data has been counted by using the formula as follows: (the certain data in 2019 – the certain data in 1990)/the certain data in 1990) × 100%. Also, all countries are divided into 5 SDI quintiles: high-, high-middle-, middle-, low-middle- and low-SDI regions, and they are also categorized into 17 GBD regions based on their different geographies. Moreover, we artificially divide these populations into 4 age groups in this paper: youth (15–44 years), middle-aged (45–59 years), middle-old-aged (60–74 years) and old-aged (75+ years); and summarize the data of each group as a new age group [16].

3. Results

3.1 Developing regions have a higher EAPC of PC-related death cases

The PC-associated health burden is showed as death cases and DALYs (YLL and YLD), and these indexes all remarkedly elevated from 1990 to 2019. Briefly,

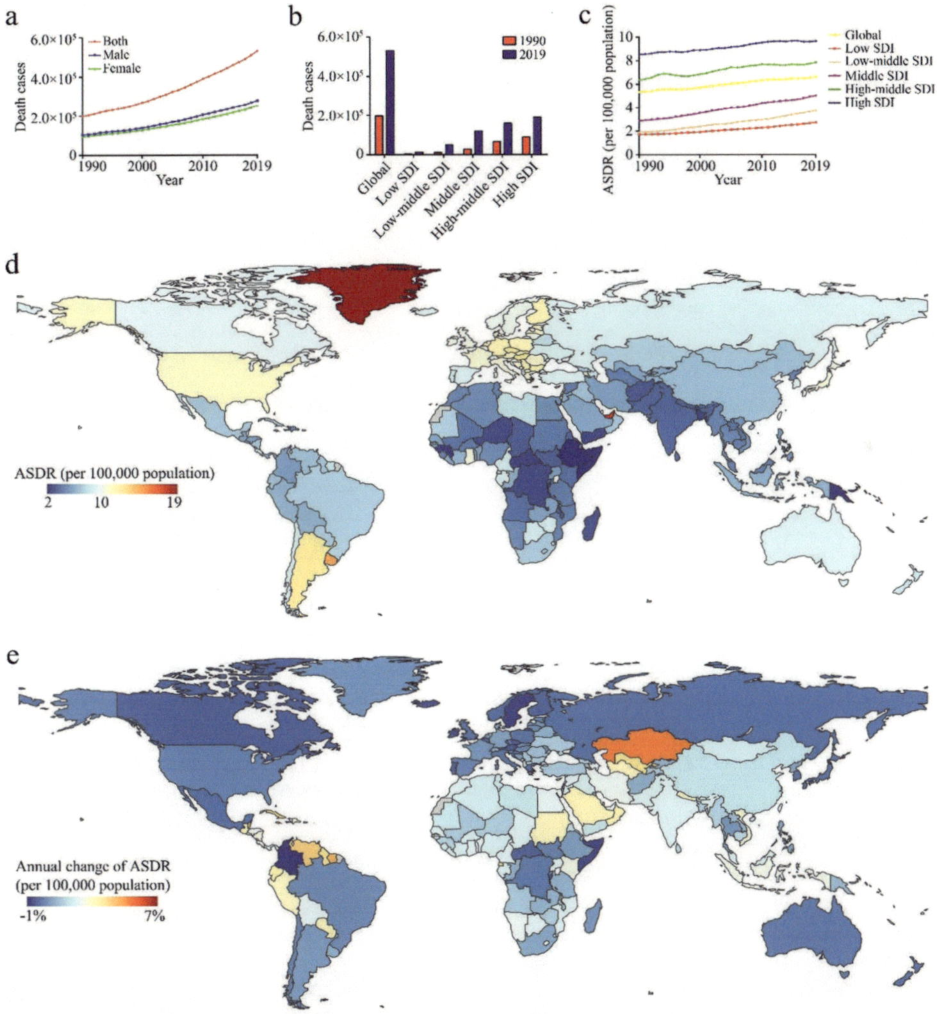

Figure 1.
Developing regions have a higher EAPC of PC-related death cases. (a) PC-related death cases at global level in 1990–2019; (b) PC-related deaths cases globally and in different SDI regions between 1990 and 2019; (c) PC-related ASDRs globally and in different SDI regions in 1990–2019; (d) PC-related ASDRs in all countries and territories from 1990 to 2019; (e) annual changes of PC-related ASDRs in all countries and territories in 1990–2019.

the total number of PC death cases ascended gradually from 0.198 million (95% uncertainty interval [UI]: 0.189–0.205) in 1990 to 0.531 million (95% UI: 0.492–0.567) in 2019 (**Figure 1a**; **Table 1**). Notably, PC-related death cases substantially up-regulated in high and high-middle SDI regions from 1990, reaching respectively 0.190 (95% UI: 0.171–0.201) and 0.160 million (95% UI: 0.146–0.171) in 2019 (**Figure 1b**; **Table 1**). Moreover, the number of DALYs ascended from 4.648 million (95% UI: 4.465–4.812) in 1990 to 11.549 million (95% UI: 10.777–12.339) in 2019, and the PC-related YLL and YLD incidence and prevalence also significantly increased as similar as DALYs (**Figure 1a** and **b**). PC is still a tumor worthy of special attention around the world, especially in the developed regions. However, the change in disease-associated deaths may result in the alteration of

	1990		2019		1990–2019
Characteristics	**Number of deaths (95% UI)**	**ASDR per 100,000 (95% UI)**	**Number of deaths (95% UI)**	**ASDR per 100,000 (95% UI)**	**EAPC of ASDR**
Global	198,050.9 (189,328.9–204,762.6)	5.337988 (5.066576–5.521704)	531,107.1 (491,948.2–566,536.9)	6.617711 (6.114269–7.062683)	0.008
Sex					
Males	103,311.8 (98,381.2–108,763.8)	6.117671 (5.811734–6.418189)	278,173.5 (257,504.9–298,745)	7.549512 (7.00679–8.093687)	0.008
Females	94,739.13 (89,322.34–98,183.68)	4.638661 (4.341669–4.816422)	252,933.6 (225,846.2–273,819.7)	5.765981 (5.149236–6.242311)	0.007
Sociodemographic index					
Low	3732.25 (2986.98–4466.39	1.706752811 (1.354595014–2.043574753)	12,945.68 (11,335.87–14,668.86)	2.719237 (2.382481–3.088279)	0.017
Low-middle	10,534.08 (8989.17–11,991.20)	1.912891 (1.620578–2.179905)	48,531.94 (44,310.31–53,080.10)	3.753841 (3.436528–4.087937)	0.024
Middle	27,839.57 (25,926.03–29,774.69)	2.873963 (2.681809–3.060948)	120,021.02 (107,034.53–134,529.10)	5.028165 (4.481748–5.633189)	0.020
High-middle	66,078.52 (63,329.31–68,573.69)	6.368478 (6.085345–6.608387)	159,583.34 (146,076.68–170,901.98)	7.842302 (7.173386–8.404491)	0.007
High	89,795.20 (85,585.16–91,855.04)	8.523968428 (8.120608505–8.7211042)	189,782.35 (171,237.17–200,954.96)	9.642343 (8.829988–10.15834)	0.005
Region					
African Union	6495.03 (5660.48–7273.16)	2.470063 (2.146529–2.789471)	24,507.33 (21,894.36–27,722.39)	4.269341 (3.833127–4.795673)	0.018
Central Europe, Eastern Europe, and Central Asia	32,988.71 (31,723.09–34,386.87-)	6.995463 (6.710744–7.293639)	55,073.43 (50,226.10–59,699.96)	8.736954 (7.972693–9.458667)	0.006

	1990		2019		1990–2019
Characteristics	**Number of deaths (95% UI)**	**ASDR per 100,000 (95% UI)**	**Number of deaths (95% UI)**	**ASDR per 100,000 (95% UI)**	**EAPC of ASDR**
Commonwealth	24,090.01 (22,069.40–25,875.86)	3.33998 (3.068543–3.58272)	76,609.06 (70,607.06–82,887.01)	4.269969 (3.921841–4.613284)	0.008
European Union	59,527.67 (57,110.58–60,782.32)	8.566903 (8.216116–8.749479)	108,799.82 (99,209.44–115,700.88)	9.904503 (9.161547–10.47891)	0.006
Four World Regions	197,890.67 (189,177.16–204,596.72)	5.342123 (5.070414–5.52598)	530,364.46 (491,286.88–565,716.10)	6.618569 (6.115779–7.063628)	0.008
G20	172,093.47 (164,304.22–177,507.19)	6.004115 (5.6873–6.205645)	440,507.51 (407,220.42–469,488.84)	7.126603 (6.569833–7.599675)	0.006
High-income	104,195.34 (99,468.66–106,572.21)	8.606354 (8.21392–8.801198)	213,898.08 (193,069.89–225,910.35)	9.691574 (8.905589–10.17949)	0.005
Latin America and Caribbean	9087.31 (8727.74–9322.18)	4.328772 (4.126848–4.454814)	33,958.87 (30,743.65–37,037.14)	5.900684 (5.338953–6.435645)	0.010
Nordic Region	3577.05 (3395.57–3691.19)	9.326386 (8.866859–9.612517)	5503.46 (5032.12–5862.14)	9.634676 (8.902379–10.24815)	0.001
North Africa and Middle East	4593.99 (3889.31–5424.34)	2.839286 (2.373719–3.362284)	22,277.14 (19,357.44–25,691.38)	5.491246 (4.784293–6.309636)	0.024
OECD Countries	113,507.83 (108,274.30–116,056.64)	8.515677 (8.115832–8.711694)	234,652.44 (212,197.36–248,342.99)	9.515365 (8.752035–10.0171)	0.004
South Asia	7736.11 (6242.63–9124.89)	1.524468 (1.21814–1.814484)	40,012.02 (35,017.30–45,582.35)	3.039063 (2.650421–3.451983)	0.024
Southeast Asia, East Asia, and Oceania	34,369.13 (30,550.47–38,437.22)	3.146132 (2.806709–3.483381)	148,207.46 (129,127.02–169,171.49)	5.676818 (4.950982–6.466765)	0.022
Sub-Saharan Africa	5080.33 (4372.88–5745.32)	2.610513 (2.238488–2.971409)	17,680.11 (15,687.82–19,936.27)	4.251351 (3.798545–4.736339)	0.016
WHO region	197,567.19 (188,860.68–204,272.86)	5.342985 (5.070932–5.527481)	529,380.03 (490,437.58–564,548.47)	6.62151 (6.119083–7.067508)	0.008
World Bank Income Levels	197,979.05 (189,259.93–204,688.94)	5.338855 (5.06738–5.522642)	530,862.92 (491,721.96–566,270.72)	6.618082 (6.114564–7.063045)	0.008
World Bank Regions	197,855.78 (189,125.74–204,570.94)	5.338191 (5.066414–5.521968)	530,520.51 (491,420.33–565,885.29)	6.616384 (6.113325–7.061656)	0.008

Table 1.
The death cases and age-standardized death rates of PC in 1990 and 2019, and their temporal trends from 1990 to 2019.

overall disease burden. The value of ASDR progressively increased (5.338 [95% UI: 5.522–5.067] per 100,000 population in 1990 and 6.618 [95% UI: 6.114–7.063] per 100,000 population in 2019 at the global level during the past three decades; and the estimated annual percentage change (EAPC) is 0.008 (**Figure 1c**; **Table 1**). In addition, EPAC of PC-related ASDR respectively is 0.005, 0.007, 0.020, 0.024, and 0.017 in high, high-middle, middle, middle-low and low SDI regions, which suggested that the EPAC of PC burden in developing regions had exceeded that in developed regions during the past 30 years.

As shown in **Table 1**, we found that PC-related death cases and ASDRs remarkedly ascended from 1900 to 2019 in most GBD regions. Briefly, the relatively high SDI regions including the European Union (9.904503 [95% UI: 9.161547–10.47891]), high-income (9.691574 [95% UI: 8.905589–10.17949]), the Nordic region (9.634676 [95% UI: 8.902379–10.24815]) and OECD countries (9.515365 [95% UI: 8.752035–10.0171]) have higher ASDR. Furthermore, ASDRs of PC increased in all GBD regions, with the maximum increase being surveyed in North Africa and Middle East (EAPC = 0.024), followed by South Asia (EAPC = 0.024), Southeast Asia, East Asia, and Oceania (EAPC = 0.022). However, relatively high SDI regions, such as the Nordic region (0.001), OECD countries (0.004) and high-income (0.005), have the lowest EAPC with higher ASDR. An extremely high ASDR was observed in Greenland (19.29 [95% UI: 15.73–22.84]), and its value was far ahead of that in other countries. On the contrary, the lowest ASDRs were found in Ethiopia, Somalia, and Papua New Guinea, with rates of 1–2 per 100,000 population in 2019 (**Figure 1d**). At the country level, Cabo verde (7.45%), Grenada (5.85%), Kazakhstan (5.74%), Dominica (5.23%), and Saint Kitts and Nevis (5.17%) had the most pronounced increases in ADSR. Interestingly, ASDRs of some developed countries in Northern Europe dropped slightly from 1990 to 2019, although most countries have obvious increases in ASDRs. For instance, Colombia, Sweden, Somalia, Iceland, and Ireland had marked decreases in ASDR; their annal percent changes are −0.54%, −0.36%, −0.29%, −0.27%, and −0.25%). As the largest developing country, current ASDR in China is 5.99 [95% UI: 5.12–6.93], with a relatively high increase in annal percent change of ASDR (2.02%) (**Figure 1e**).

3.2 Sex differences in PC-related burden may further decrease

As shown in **Table 1**, PC-associated death cases at the global level significantly up-regulated in both males and females from 1990 to 2019, and it respectively reached 0.278 (95% UI: 0.258–0.299) million in males and 0.253 (95% CI: 0.226–0.274) million in females in 2019, which also showed that men had incessantly higher mortality than women in PC burden. Similarly, males had higher ASDRs than females, and the highest (males *vs*. females = 11.099390 *vs*. 8.307626) and lowest (males *vs*. females = 2.946914 *vs*. 2.499140) ASDRs were separately found in high and low SDI regions (**Figure 2a**). It is worth noting that the ASDR alterations in women increased more notably than in men during the past three decades in "Low SDI" and "Low-middle SDI" regions (**Figure 2b**), resulting in decreases in the ASDR ratio of men to women, and they had reached approximately 1.18 and 1.10, respectively, in 2019 (**Figure 2c**). In the 17 GBD regions, ASDR of male outweighed that of female in most regions except the Nordic region (**Figure 2d**). Males had higher PC death cases than females with diminishing differences in sex, and thereby, the higher increase of PC-related deaths in females is a matter worthy of attention, especially in developing regions.

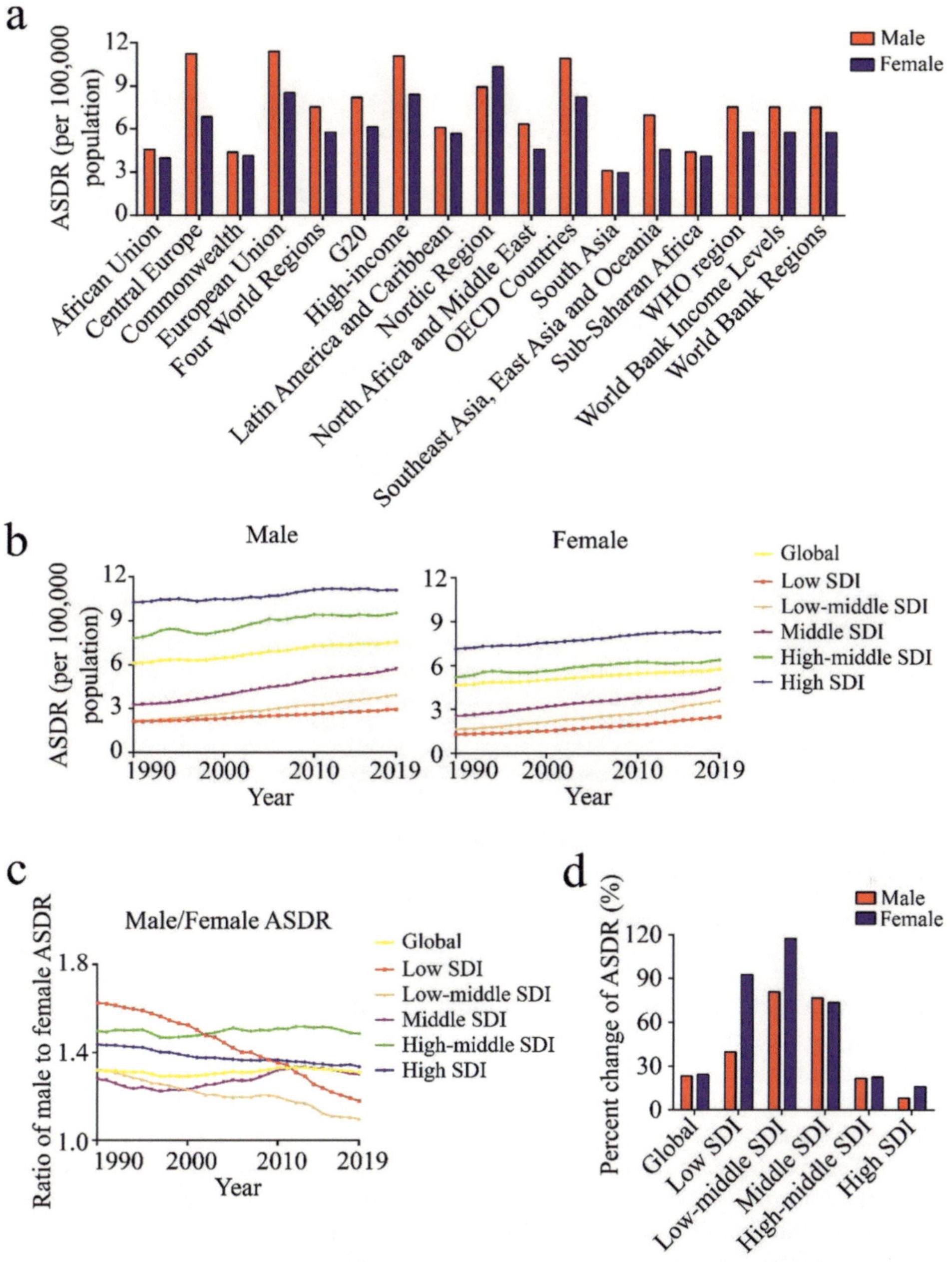

Figure 2.
Sex differences in PC-related burden may further decrease. (a) PC-related ASDRs in males and females globally and in different SDI regions in 1990–2019; (b) percent changes of PC-related ASDRs in males and females globally and in different SDI regions between 1990 and 2019; (c) the ratios of male to female globally and in different SDI regions in 1990–2019; (d) PC-related ASDRs in males and females globally and in 17 GBD SDI regions between 1990 and 2019.

3.3 Developing regions have a higher rate of premature death in PC

Figure 3a illustrates that PC-related deaths tended to increase with age, with the 65–69, 70–74, 65–69, 70–74, and 75–79 age populations having the highest death

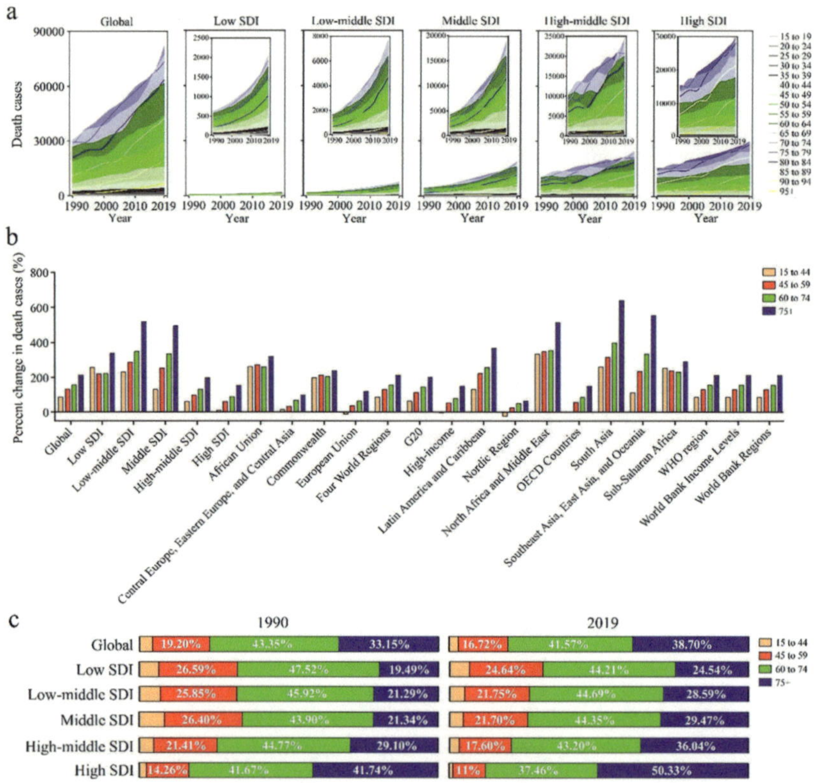

Figure 3.
Developing regions have a higher rate of premature death in PC. (a) the distribution of PC-related death cases at different age groups globally and in different SDI regions from 1990 to 2019; (b) percent changes in PC-related death cases in four age groups between 1990 and 2019 globally and in different SDI regions; (c) percentages of PC-related death cares at four age groups globally and in different SDI regions between 1990 and 2019.

cases in low, low-middle, middle, high-middle, and high SDI regions, respectively. Moreover, we artificially divided these populations into different age groups: youth, middle-aged, middle-old-aged and old-aged; and then analyzed each group's respective death rates in every SDI region and compared them. At the global level, there was the greatest up-regulation in death cases in the old-aged populations from 1990 to 2019 (**Figure 3b**). As a result, the number of deaths in 75+ groups increased more rapidly in low-middle SDI regions between 1990 and 2019 than in other SDI regions, as well as the number of youth deaths in low SDI regions increased faster than in other SDI regions. On the contrary, death cases in some developed regions, such as European Union, High-income and the Nordic region, had obvious declines in the youth groups from 1990 to 2019 (**Figure 3b**). In addition, a trend toward older ages was evident in the population who died from PC-associated causes from 1990 to 2019, and there were more elderly individuals who died from PC in high SDI regions than in low SDI regions (**Figure 3c**). According to data from 1990 and 2019, low SDI regions had the youngest distribution of PC-related deaths, and the proportions of patients under 60 years were 33% and 31% in 1990 and 2019, respectively. By comparison, the age distribution of death rates for PC-related deaths was the highest for high SDI regions, with elderly individuals accounting for 42% in 1990 and 50% in 2019. Accordingly, deaths related to PC in developing regions are not only increasing faster than those in developed regions but also affecting younger populations (at ages 15–44 years), which is a relatively serious problem.

3.4 The burden of PC death is partly due to the poor control of smoking, FPG, and BMI

As shown in **Figure 4a**, the risk factors including high metabolic risk factors (BMI and FPG) and behavioral risk factor (smoking) attributable to ASDRs of PC changed by 51.6%, 66.9%, and – 1.00%, respectively, from 1990 to 2019. The smoking risk factor, however, remained the leading cause of ASDR increase in 2019, and it was also the top factor contributing to ASDRs in all SDI regions. Smoking-related mortality has declined substantially in high SDI countries, but it remains an important risk factor

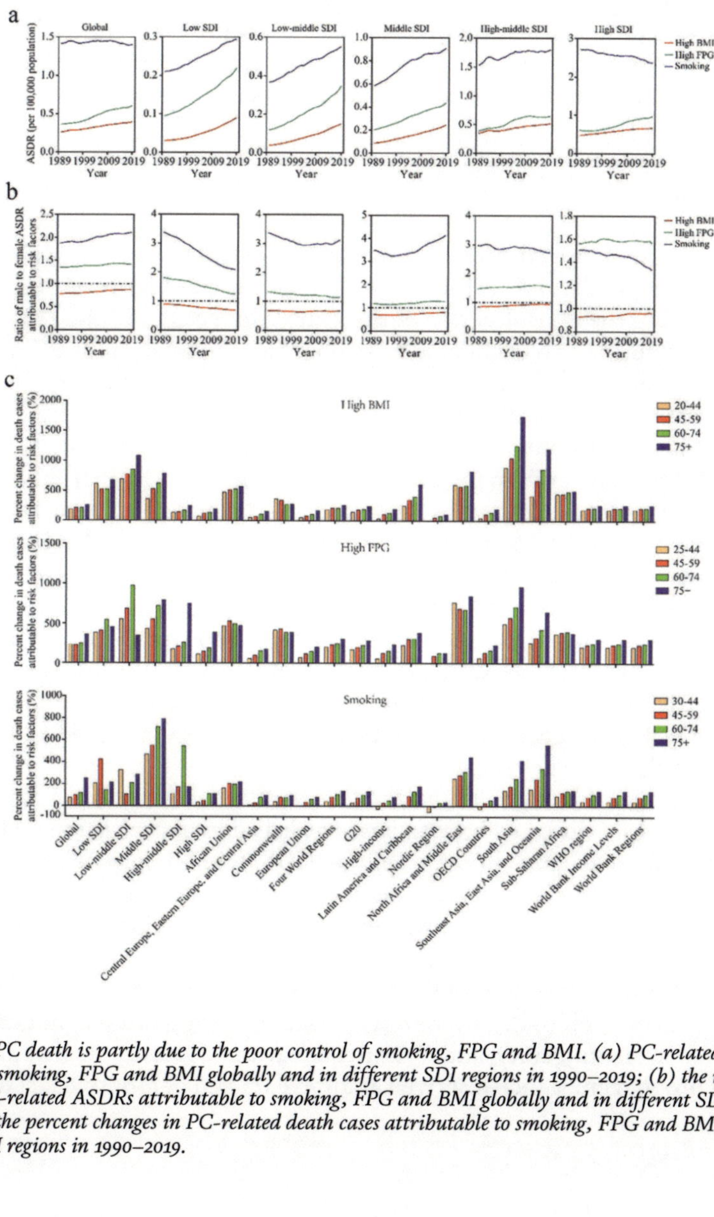

Figure 4.
The burden of PC death is partly due to the poor control of smoking, FPG and BMI. (a) PC-related ASDRs attributable to smoking, FPG and BMI globally and in different SDI regions in 1990–2019; (b) the ratios of male to female of PC-related ASDRs attributable to smoking, FPG and BMI globally and in different SDI regions in 1990–2019; (c) the percent changes in PC-related death cases attributable to smoking, FPG and BMI globally and in different SDI regions in 1990–2019.

with a high ASDR value of 2.37 per 100,000 in 2019. In contrast, ASDRs attributable to high BMI and FPG significantly increased in all SDI regions. Smoking and high FPG risk factors contributed to the higher ASDR among men than women worldwide. For smoking, the sex ratio (male to female) was greater than 1.8, suggesting that this risk was still a key contributing factor to the differences in PC-caused death rates. The smoking risk factor was associated with a significant decline in deaths in other SDI regions across all age groups; however, an increase in this parameter was observed in the middle SDI region over the same period (**Figure 4b**). At the geographical level, developing regions including North Africa, Middle East, South Asia, Southeast Asia, East Asia, and Oceania exhibited the fastest growth in high BMI and FPG-attributed death rates at all ages (**Figure 4c**). In sharp contrast, developed regions, such as the Nordic region, OECD countries, and high-income regions showed minimal increases. As a result, metabolic risk factors pose major challenges to reducing PC-related deaths throughout the world, but especially in developing nations. The smoking rate has declined in youth groups in the following locations: Nordic region, OECD countries, and high-income regions; and Southeast Asia, East Asia, and Oceania were the regions with the highest growth rate in PC-related death cases over this time.

4. Discussion

PC remains a high mortality disease worldwide with a 5-year survival rate of less than 10%, and metabolic risk factors and smoking tobacco have been largely responsible for increasing the mortality rate of this cancer in recent decades [19, 20]. The present study, in terms of our understanding, is the latest analysis of PC-associated burden and risk factors at the global level. Researchers have shown that the PC-caused burden is similar to the overall cancer burden trend [21, 22]. Across the world, this study found that the absolute number of PC-related deaths increased from 0.198 million in 1990 to 0.531 million in 2019. Further, the global ASDR of PC has shown a gradual increase in the past 30 years, suggesting that population increase and aging may be responsible for the up-regulation in death cases. Additionally, the ASDR trend value can serve as an indicator reflecting changes in disease patterns and risk factors, so we used the EAPC index of ASDR to reflect such changes in the last three decades [23–25]. The results showed that ASDR was up-regulated from 1990 to 2019 along with SDI's improvement; briefly, EPAC of PC-related ASDR was 0.005, 0.007, 0.020, 0.024, and 0.017 in high, high-middle, middle, middle-low, and low SDI regions, respectively. During the past three decades, developing regions have had a greater EPAC of PC burden than developed regions.

It is worth noting that high FPG and BMI as well as smoking have become the primary drivers of PC-induced burden, and the inability to manage these factors has led to an increase in the mortality rate in lower SDI regions compared to improved SDI regions. As a result of economic growth, developed regions, such as the European Union and the United States, have also seen increases in metabolic disease incidence. There has been a significant decline in the mortality rate associated with metabolic risk factors as a result of decades of strengthening health promotion guidelines in developed countries [26–28]. Moreover, tobacco smoking is the major cause of avoidable premature mortality, and it results in various diseases, such as lung, pancreatic, and oropharynx cancers, as well as apoplexia and coronary heart disease.

Importantly, smoking has gradually decreased in many developed countries due to the effective policies to combat tobacco use; but the developing countries are still at risk because of the aggressive strategies of lucrative tobacco companies [29, 30]. PC-related death cases have substantially increased over recent decades in developing regions including North Africa, Middle East, South Asia, Southeast Asia, East Asia, and Oceania. In China, for example, PC is estimated to affect over 0.117 million people in 2019. As a result of rapid economic transformation, industrialization, and urbanization in these regions, diet and lifestyle have changed significantly, which has exacerbated the rise of metabolic diseases and smoking-related diseases [31–33]. It is therefore imperative to take effective steps to slow the adverse trend in developing regions.

As part of this study, we further found that male PC deaths and ASDRs are higher than female deaths and that the gap between male and female PC deaths has decreased. In addition to biological factors, smoking risk factors and BMI may also contribute to gender-based differences [34, 35]. Smoking-related ASDRs are notably higher in males, which indicates that smoking is an important risk factor leading to gender differences in PC-caused death burden. The analysis of the ASDR ratio between men and women in high SDI regions indicates that the contribution of high FPG has exceeded smoking, which is the most important risk factor in other SDI regions. Therefore, it is necessary to increase awareness of these risk factors and improve corresponding management to further decline sex-specific differences in PC mortality. In addition, further consideration should be taken to reflect changes in the burden of PC-related deaths among populations at different life stages, and this paper thereby investigated the percentage change in death cases in four artificially divided age groups: youth, middle-aged, middle-old-aged, and old-aged. Globally, most deaths from PC are caused by people aged 60–74 years; however, the majority in high SDI region is mainly caused by people 75 years and older perhaps because of medical progress and population aging. The number of premature deaths (15–44 years) has increased significantly over the past three decades, except for in some developed areas, such as the European Union, high-income countries, and the Nordic region. Based on these opposite trends, developed and developing countries show a substantial gap in interventions aimed at reducing early mortality. Worldwide, the elderly population remains the main target in PC prevention and treatment; however, the low SDI countries should also boost their management of youths at high risk for PC.

In summary, as a consequence of rapid economic and dietary structure development in developing countries, PC has gradually become a common cancer worldwide, as well as there has been a higher increase of EAPC of PC-related deaths in developing countries. The main cause of this change is the lack of control of PC risk factors, such as FPG, BMI, and smoking in lower SDI areas. Furthermore, developing regions should also pay attention to the rapidly increasing rate of premature deaths. To reduce the number of PC-related deaths and burden, it is the most important to intervene in the early stages of PC in order to significantly decrease the risk factors. Meanwhile, compared with the developing regions, developed countries should maintain continuous efforts in reducing PC-related risks in the future. The renewal of PC burden analysis in this paper at multiple levels in GBD database is very beneficial for each country to determine individual policies to control the increasing trend of this disease.

Funding

We first appreciate the great work by the Global Burden of Disease Study 2019 collaborators. This work was supported by grants from the Research Project established by Chinese Pharmaceutical Association Hospital Pharmacy department (NO. CPA-Z05-ZC-2022-002).

Authors' contributions

X.T. designed the study and wrote the manuscript. X.T., H.X., and D.D. collected and analyzed the data. L.L. performed the statistical analysis. X.T. and H.X. edited the manuscript and provided valuable suggestions for study design and data analysis. All authors have approved the final version of this paper.

Conflict of interest

The authors declare that they have no competing interests.

Consent for publication

Not applicable

Ethics approval and consent to participate

Not applicable

Availability of data and material

The datasets used and/or analyzed during the current study are available from the corresponding author on reasonable request.

Abbreviations

PC	pancreatic cancer
FPG	fasting plasma glucose
BMI	body mass index
GBD	Global Burden of Diseases
IRFS	Injuries and Risk Factors Study
ASDR	age-standardized death rate
SDI	sociodemographic index
GHDx	Global Health Data Exchange
DALYs	disability-adjusted life years
YLLs	years of life lost
YLDs	years of life lived with disability

Appendix

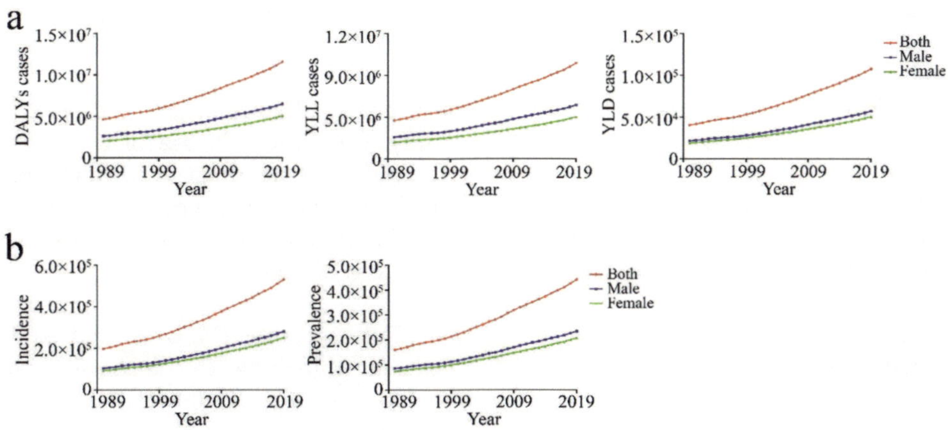

Figure A1.
(a) PC-related DALYs, YLL and YLD at global level in 1990–2019; (b) PC-related incidence and prevalence at global level in 1990–2019.

Author details

Hong Xiang[1], Deshi Dong[2], Linlin Lv[2] and Xufeng Tao[2]*

1 Laboratory of Integrative Medicine, First Affiliated Hospital of Dalian Medical University, Dalian, China

2 Department of Pharmacy, First Affiliated Hospital of Dalian Medical University, Dalian, China

*Address all correspondence to: taoxufeng.2008@163.com

References

[1] Connor AA, Gallinger S. Pancreatic cancer evolution and heterogeneity: Integrating omics and clinical data. Nature Reviews. Cancer. 2022;**22**(3):131-142

[2] Tao X, Xiang H, Pan Y, et al. Pancreatitis initiated pancreatic ductal adenocarcinoma: Pathophysiology explaining clinical evidence. Pharmacological Research. 2021;**168**:105595

[3] Carreras-Torres R, Johansson M, Gaborieau V, et al. The role of obesity, type 2 diabetes, and metabolic factors in pancreatic cancer: A Mendelian randomization study. Journal of the National Cancer Institute. 2017;**109**(9):djx012

[4] Collisson EA, Bailey P, Chang DK, Biankin AV. Molecular subtypes of pancreatic cancer. Nature Reviews. Gastroenterology & Hepatology. 2019;**16**(4):207-220

[5] Rahib L, Smith BD, Aizenberg R, Rosenzweig AB, Fleshman JM, Matrisian LM. Projecting cancer incidence and deaths to 2030: The unexpected burden of thyroid, liver, and pancreas cancers in the United States. Cancer Research. 2014;**74**(11):2913-2921

[6] Yusuf S, Joseph P, Rangarajan S, et al. Modifiable risk factors, cardiovascular disease, and mortality in 155 722 individuals from 21 high-income, middle-income, and low-income countries (PURE): A prospective cohort study. Lancet. 2020;**395**(10226):795-808

[7] Sankhla M, Sharma TK, Gahlot S, et al. The ominous link between obesity and abdominal adiposity with diabetes and diabetic dyslipidemia in diabetic population of developing country. Clinical Laboratory. 2013;**59**(1-2):155-161

[8] Martha S, Ramreddy S, Pantam N. Study of impaired glucose tolerance, dyslipidemia, metabolic syndrome, and cardiovascular risk in a south Indian population. Journal of Postgraduate Medicine. 2011;**57**(1):4-8

[9] Wipfli H, Samet JM. One hundred years in the making: The global tobacco epidemic. Annual Review of Public Health. 2016;**37**:149-166

[10] Yang JJ, Yu D, Wen W, et al. Tobacco smoking and mortality in Asia: A pooled Meta-analysis. JAMA Network Open. 2019;**2**(3):e191474

[11] GBD 2017 Pancreatic Cancer Collaborators. The global, regional, and national burden of pancreatic cancer and its attributable risk factors in 195 countries and territories, 1990-2017: Global burden of 87 risk factors for the Global Burden of Disease Study 2017. Lancet Gastroenterology Hepatology. 2019;**4**(12):934-947

[12] Huang J, Lok V, Ngai CH, et al. Worldwide burden of, risk factors for, and trends in pancreatic Cancer. Gastroenterology. 2021;**160**(3):744-754

[13] GBD 2013 Mortality and Causes of Death Collaborators. Global, regional, and national age-sex specific all-cause and cause-specific mortality for 240 causes of death, 1990-2013: A systematic analysis for the Global Burden of Disease Study 2013. Lancet. 2015;**385**(9963):117-171

[14] GBD 2019 Diseases and Injuries Collaborators. Global burden of 369 diseases and injuries in 204

countries and territories, 1990-2019: A systematic analysis for the Global Burden of Disease Study 2019. Lancet. 2020;**396**(10258):1204-1222

[15] GBD 2019 Risk Factors Collaborators. Global burden of 87 risk factors in 204 countries and territories, 1990-2019: A systematic analysis for the Global Burden of Disease Study 2019. Lancet. 2020;**396**(10258):1223-1249

[16] Wang W, Hu M, Liu H, et al. Global Burden of Disease Study 2019 suggests that metabolic risk factors are the leading drivers of the burden of ischemic heart disease. Cell Metabolism. 2021;**33**(10):1943-1956.e2

[17] Hankey BF, Ries LA, Kosary CL, et al. Partitioning linear trends in age-adjusted rates. Cancer Causes & Control. 2000;**11**(1):31-35

[18] Rahib L, Wehner MR, Matrisian LM, Nead KT. Estimated projection of US Cancer incidence and death to 2040. JAMA Network Open. 2021;**4**(4):e214708

[19] Mizrahi JD, Surana R, Valle JW, Shroff RT. Pancreatic cancer. Lancet. 2020;**395**(10242):2008-2020

[20] Park W, Chawla A, O'Reilly EM. Pancreatic cancer: A review. Journal of the American Medical Association. 2021;**326**(9):851-862

[21] Global Burden of Disease Cancer Collaboration, Fitzmaurice C, Abate D, et al. Global, Regional, and National Cancer Incidence, mortality, years of life lost, years lived with disability, and disability-adjusted life-years for 29 cancer groups, 1990 to 2017: A systematic analysis for the global burden of disease study. JAMA Oncologia. 2019;**5**(12):1749-1768

[22] Mattiuzzi C, Lippi G. Cancer statistics: A comparison between World Health Organization (WHO) and global burden of disease (GBD). European Journal of Public Health. 2020;**30**(5):1026-1027

[23] Chen MM, Zhang X, Liu YM, et al. Heavy disease burden of high systolic blood pressure during 1990-2019: Highlighting regional, sex, and age specific strategies in blood pressure control. Frontier in Cardiovascular Medicine. 2021;**8**:754778

[24] Hung GY, Horng JL, Yen HJ, Lee CY, Lin LY. Changing incidence patterns of hepatocellular carcinoma among age groups in Taiwan. Journal of Hepatology. 2015;**63**(6):1390-1396

[25] Liu Z, Jiang Y, Yuan H, et al. The trends in incidence of primary liver cancer caused by specific etiologies: Results from the global burden of disease study 2016 and implications for liver cancer prevention. Journal of Hepatology. 2019;**70**(4):674-683

[26] Opio J, Croker E, Odongo GS, Attia J, Wynne K, McEvoy M. Metabolically healthy overweight/obesity are associated with increased risk of cardiovascular disease in adults, even in the absence of metabolic risk factors: A systematic review and meta-analysis of prospective cohort studies. Obesity Reviews. 2020;**21**(12):e13127

[27] Blüher M. Metabolically healthy obesity. Endocrine Reviews. 2020;**41**(3):bnaa004

[28] Chow CK, Teo KK, Rangarajan S, et al. Prevalence, awareness, treatment, and control of hypertension in rural and urban communities in high-, middle-, and low-income countries. Journal of the American Medical Association. 2013;**310**(9):959-968

[29] Samet JM. Tobacco smoking: The leading cause of preventable disease

worldwide. Thoracic Surgery Clinics. 2013;**23**(2):103-112

[30] Britton J. Progress with the global tobacco epidemic. Lancet. 2015;**385**(9972):924-926

[31] Bandosz P, O'Flaherty M, Drygas W, et al. Decline in mortality from coronary heart disease in Poland after socioeconomic transformation: Modelling study. BMJ. 2012;**344**:d8136

[32] Du S, Lü B, Wang Z, Zhai F. Transition of dietary pattern in China. Wei Sheng Yan Jiu. 2001;**30**(4):221-225

[33] Tian Y, Jiang C, Wang M, et al. BMI, leisure-time physical activity, and physical fitness in adults in China: Results from a series of national surveys, 2000-14. The Lancet Diabetes and Endocrinology. 2016;**4**(6):487-497

[34] Ferndale L, Aldous C, Hift R, Thomson S. Gender differences in oesophageal squamous cell carcinoma in a South African tertiary hospital. International Journal of Environmental Research and Public Health. 2020;**17**(19):7086

[35] GBD 2016 Causes of Death Collaborators. Global, regional, and national age-sex specific mortality for 264 causes of death, 1980-2016: A systematic analysis for the Global Burden of Disease Study 2016. Lancet. 2017;**390**(10100):1151-1210

Chapter 2

Managing Risk Factors in the Emergency Department

Rafael Suárez del Villar Carrero

Abstract

This chapter aims to provide a comprehensive guide for healthcare professionals on addressing and managing key risk factors associated with chronic and acute illnesses in emergency care settings. The emergency department often serves as a critical juncture where timely identification of risk factors can significantly influence patient outcomes. The scope of the chapter includes commonly encountered risk factors such as hypertension, diabetes, smoking, alcoholism, and obesity. It offers insights into rapid assessment tools like risk scales and quick lab tests that are practical for an emergency setting. Additionally, the chapter will explore evidence-based interventions for immediate stabilization and risk factor management, emphasizing the need for interdisciplinary coordination. Effective communication strategies for healthcare providers to use with both colleagues and patients will also be discussed. The chapter concludes with recommendations for implementing up-to-date protocols and emphasizes the need for ongoing professional training.

Keywords: emergency department, risk factors, management, chronic disease, acute disease

1. Introduction

The environment of the emergency department (ED) is uniquely dynamic and unpredictable, which inherently carries high risks. During a shift, ED personnel may face a wide range of situations, ranging from common cold cases to critical situations of trauma or cardiac arrest demanding intensive resuscitation efforts. In this context, agile decision-making is necessary, understood as the ability to make informed and timely decisions in an environment where every second counts. This highlights the need for speed, efficiency, and accuracy in the assessment, diagnosis, and treatment of patients [1].

Proper management of clinical risk factors is essential in this setting, especially due to the often-overwhelming flow of patients. This management involves the identification, evaluation, and control of risks associated with medical care in the ED, including the risks of infections, medication errors, and other complications that may arise. Effective management of these risks can not only make a significant difference in the clinical evolution of patients, aiding in avoiding major complications and promoting a quicker recovery, but can also result in a notable reduction of costs associated with medical care. Complications arising from poor management of risk factors can generate a considerable economic burden due to extended hospitalizations, additional treatments, and additional resources needed to address these complications. Therefore, adequate risk management is essential not only from a clinical perspective but also an economic one, contributing to the optimization of available resources and the sustainability of the healthcare system [2].

Various researchers have highlighted methodologies in risk management in emergency medicine. A palpable example is the early identification of sepsis, a critical condition that can be fatal if not treated promptly. The implementation of sepsis protocols, such as the rapid administration of antibiotics and fluids, is essential in these cases [3]. Additionally, effective management of patients with chronic diseases, such as diabetes or heart disease, is crucial to avoid complications arising from hyperglycemic or hypoglycemic crises, where early intervention can prevent severe complications and improve outcomes [4, 5].

In the ED, every decision and action have immediate and long-term implications on the patient's health. The identification and adequate management of risk factors, such as pre-existing chronic diseases or acute symptoms, are essential to provide effective and safe care [2]. The management of these factors goes beyond the treatment of the presented conditions; it includes the anticipation and mitigation of possible complications. Effective risk management requires a systematic approach that allows for accurate documentation and treatment of the patient, minimizing unexpected errors and thus improving patient outcomes in this critical environment [6].

The dynamics in this Department are unique, with a fast pace and crucial decisions made within a very short span. Each patient entering the doors represents a set of risks that need to be evaluated and managed effectively to ensure appropriate and timely treatment. Interaction with the patient in the ED is a critical opportunity to identify and address risk factors that could adversely affect their health, both in the short and long term. A proactive approach to risk management can facilitate a smooth transition of the patient towards a complete recovery and reduce the likelihood of readmissions. For instance, effective communication between ED personnel and the patient, along with proper follow-up upon discharge, can help manage risks more effectively and improve patient satisfaction [7]. This communication can include clear explanations of diagnoses, treatments, and steps to follow discharge, as well as establishing an open channel of communication for any queries or concerns that may arise later.

2. Risk factors in the emergency department

2.1 Patient inherent risk factors

In the emergency department, effectively managing patient-specific risk factors is key to providing personalized medical care and forecasting clinical outcomes. These factors encompass a broad spectrum, including preexisting health conditions and psychosocial attributes, each playing a significant role in patient assessment and treatment strategies.

At the outset of discussing risk factors in the ED, it's beneficial to refer to **Table 1**, which provides a concise overview of common risk factors encountered in this setting. Chronic illnesses such as diabetes and heart disease are particularly impactful in emergency settings. For instance, a diabetic patient may present with a

Risk Factor	Prevalence	Warning Signs	Initial Management Strategies
Hypertension	Very common	Elevated blood pressure, headache	Blood pressure measurement, administration of antihypertensives
Diabetes	Common	High/low blood sugar levels, excessive thirst, fatigue	Glucose monitoring, administration of insulin or hypoglycemics
Heart Diseases	Common	Chest pain, shortness of breath, fatigue	ECG, administration of heart medications, oxygen
Trauma	Variable	Visible injuries, pain, bleeding	Stabilization, pain management, blood loss prevention
Acute Infections	Common	Fever, chills, signs of infection	Cultures, antibiotics, fluid support
Pulmonary Disease	Moderately common	Cough, difficulty breathing, wheezing	Pulse oximetry, bronchodilators, steroids

ECG: Electrocardiogram; BP: blood pressure.

Table 1.
Common risk factors in the emergency department.

life-threatening hyperglycemic crisis, necessitating immediate intervention and careful ongoing glucose monitoring. Understanding a patient's comprehensive medical history, including previous surgeries, allergies, and current medications, is vital to prevent adverse drug interactions and to fully grasp their health status. For example, a patient with a history of allergic reactions to certain antibiotics will require alternative treatment options.

Age-specific considerations are also crucial. Pediatric patients may present with symptoms that differ significantly from adults, like fever in a child potentially indicating a more severe infection. Similarly, elderly patients often have multiple comorbidities, making them more susceptible to adverse reactions from standard emergency treatments.

Psychosocial and behavioral elements play a pivotal role in medical management. A patient experiencing high stress or anxiety levels, for instance, might exhibit heightened pain sensitivity or have a panic attack, mimicking more serious conditions like myocardial infarction. Substance use can further complicate diagnosis and treatment, as in the case of an intoxicated patient who might require a different approach to pain management or may not accurately report symptoms.

Finally, individual physiological responses and genetic predispositions are key considerations. A patient with a genetic predisposition to clotting disorders, for example, might require a different approach to managing a suspected deep vein thrombosis. Such personalized health variations call for tailored diagnostic and treatment strategies to ensure effective and compassionate care in the ED.

2.2 Environmental risk factors

In the emergency department, environmental factors play a critical role in determining the quality and effectiveness of medical care. A primary challenge is managing patient overload, which often leads to extended waiting times and can delay urgent treatments. This issue not only tests the staff's ability to manage patient flow efficiently but also impacts the timeliness of care delivery.

The availability of key resources, such as essential medications and medical equipment, directly affects treatment capabilities. Limited resources can constrain treatment options, leading to delays in care provision. Equally important is the staffing level in the ED. Both the number of staff and their level of training are crucial; shortages or lack of adequate training can compromise the quality of care provided.

The physical layout and infrastructure of the ED also significantly influence care delivery. An effectively designed ED can enhance workflow, increase efficiency, and improve patient safety. Conversely, poor design may impede effective care delivery and compromise safety. Additionally, the work environment in the ED, often marked by high stress and chaos, can affect both staff decision-making abilities and their capacity to focus on patient-centered care.

Effective health information systems are essential for ensuring efficient communication and coordination of patient care. These systems facilitate the sharing of critical patient information among healthcare professionals, aiding in more informed decision-making.

Lastly, strict adherence to safety protocols and infection prevention measures is paramount in maintaining a safe environment for both patients and staff. For example, during the COVID-19 pandemic, EDs that implemented rigorous infection control measures, such as separate triage areas for suspected cases, effectively minimized cross-infection risks.

2.3 Clinical risk factors

In emergency medicine, effective decision-making and treatment hinge on recognizing and managing clinical risk factors. These include the presentation of acute symptoms and potential complications during medical care. For instance, symptoms like chest pain or breathing difficulties demand immediate assessment as they may signal life-threatening conditions. A prompt and accurate diagnosis is essential to prevent inappropriate treatments and mitigate the risk of adverse outcomes.

In the emergency department, treatment complications such as adverse drug reactions or problems arising from invasive procedures can significantly elevate clinical risks. A case in point is the management of a heart attack, stroke, or sepsis, where rapid and accurate intervention is critical. Such situations underscore the importance of vigilant monitoring and strict adherence to established medical protocols. Moreover, coordinating with various medical specialties is key in providing comprehensive and effective treatment.

Additionally, managing the risk of infectious disease transmission is a paramount concern in the ED. Implementing strict infection control measures, including proper isolation procedures, is crucial in preventing the spread of infections to both patients and healthcare staff. This aspect was particularly highlighted during the COVID-19 pandemic, where EDs worldwide adapted their protocols to manage the heightened risk of virus transmission.

Overall, managing clinical risk factors in the ED is a dynamic and critical aspect of emergency medical care, essential for ensuring patient safety and achieving optimal clinical outcomes.

2.4 Communication risk factors

Effective communication in the emergency department (ED) is crucial for delivering high-quality care. Miscommunication can lead to incorrect clinical decisions or treatment delays, especially during critical times such as shift changes or patient transfers.

For instance, consider a scenario where a patient's allergy information is inaccurately communicated during a shift change, leading to an avoidable adverse reaction. This highlights the importance of clear, concise, and accurate information transfer among healthcare professionals.

Communicating with patients and their families is equally important. Providing clear explanations about diagnoses, treatment options, and care plans is vital for informed consent and treatment adherence. Effective communication in these areas not only aids in medical decision-making but also helps alleviate patient and family anxiety, boosting overall satisfaction.

Handling sensitive situations, such as delivering difficult news or discussing end-of-life care, requires empathy, respect, and clear communication. This aspect of communication is critical for maintaining trust and providing compassionate care.

Developing communication skills among ED staff is therefore essential. Regular training sessions, role-playing scenarios, and feedback mechanisms can help staff enhance these skills. Additionally, implementing clear communication guidelines and utilizing efficient health information systems can play a significant role in mitigating communication-related risks. For example, electronic health records that are easily accessible and updateable can ensure that critical patient information is accurately recorded and shared.

2.5 Systemic risk factors

Structural and organizational elements play a pivotal role in the quality and safety of emergency care. These elements include the implementation of evidence-based protocols and effective coordination among various medical services. The absence of standardized protocols can lead to variability in patient care, compromising both quality and safety. Consistently applied, evidence-based protocols ensure that staff across the board manage emergencies effectively, adhering to the best current practices.

One case illustrating the importance of protocol standardization involved a large urban ED that implemented a new stroke protocol. This protocol streamlined the process for identifying stroke symptoms, expedited imaging, and facilitated faster treatment decisions. As a result, the department saw a notable reduction in door-to-treatment times for stroke patients.

Effective coordination within the ED and with other hospital units is another critical factor. Poor coordination can lead to delayed treatments and negatively affect patient outcomes. An example of improved coordination can be seen in a regional hospital where the introduction of an integrated patient transfer system reduced wait times and improved patient flow, directly impacting the quality of care and patient satisfaction.

The integration of health information systems is essential for systemic risk management. These systems improve communication among healthcare professionals, ensure the accuracy of patient records, and enhance the efficiency of workflows. They provide quick, reliable access to patient information, crucial for making informed decisions in high-pressure situations. For instance, an ED adopted an advanced electronic health record system, which led to improved patient tracking, reduced medication errors, and enhanced overall treatment efficiency.

Adapting rapidly to the evolving needs of the ED, particularly during public health crises or disasters, is vital for efficient and safe care delivery. An example of this adaptability was seen during a recent pandemic when an ED quickly expanded its capacity and implemented new infection control protocols, effectively managing the surge in patient volume while maintaining safety standards.

3. Methodologies and tools for risk Management in the emergency department

In the emergency department, where situations change rapidly and unpredictably, the implementation of robust risk management methodologies and tools is critical. These strategies enable swift and precise patient assessments and foster effective responses to critical conditions. This section examines widely used methodologies and cutting-edge tools that bolster effective risk management and how their implementation can elevate patient outcomes and enhance operational efficiency.

3.1 Risk assessment methodologies

3.1.1 Triage systems

Triage systems like the Emergency Severity Index (ESI), **Figure 1**, are pivotal in assessing patient acuity and determining treatment priorities. These systems aid in categorizing patients based on the severity of their conditions, ensuring that those in most need receive immediate care. Recent studies, such as the one featured in the

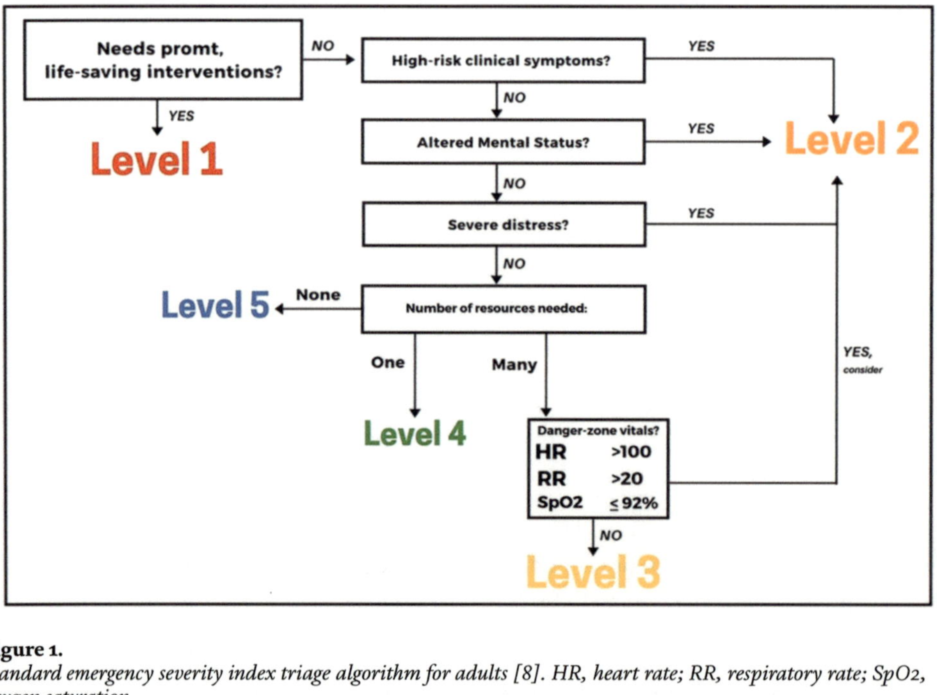

Figure 1.
Standard emergency severity index triage algorithm for adults [8]. HR, heart rate; RR, respiratory rate; SpO2, oxygen saturation.

Scandinavian Journal of Trauma, Resuscitation and Emergency Medicine, highlight how the implementation of such triage systems has led to improved patient outcomes in specific emergency situations like trauma, stroke, sepsis, and acute coronary syndrome. These findings underline the crucial role of triage systems in not only streamlining patient flow but also in significantly enhancing the quality of care and patient safety in emergency settings [9].

3.1.2 Clinical decision rules

Tools like the Ottawa Ankle Rules or the HEART Score for chest pain evaluation guide clinicians in making evidence-based decisions, thereby reducing unnecessary diagnostics while ensuring patient safety. These decision rules, as part of systematic approaches to assessment and risk management, have been instrumental in the effective identification and management of clinical deterioration in the ED. The same study emphasizes that systematic methods following initial triage assessments have emerged over the last decade, significantly contributing to the recognition of deteriorating patients and establishing standards for expected responses [10]. This systematic approach to risk assessment and management aligns with the global priority of enhancing patient safety in emergency care.

By integrating these methodologies and utilizing data from extensive studies, the ED can significantly improve its capability to manage risks, leading to better patient outcomes and heightened operational efficiency. These strategies are not only vital for addressing immediate patient needs but also play a crucial role in fortifying a more structured and reliable emergency care system.

3.2 Data-driven tools

3.2.1 Predictive analytics

Utilizing data analytics to forecast patterns in patient influx, identify high-risk cases, and predict resource needs. For instance, analyzing historical data to predict peak times helps in resource allocation, thus reducing wait times and improving patient throughput.

3.2.2 Electronic health records (EHR)

EHR systems play a vital role in centralizing patient information, enhancing provider communication, and allowing swift access to crucial patient data. These systems improve documentation, facilitate better care coordination, and support decision-making.

3.3 Technology-enhanced tools

3.3.1 Telemedicine

Platforms for telemedicine can speed up consultations with specialists, particularly valuable in remote or understaffed EDs. They broaden patient access to expert care and are pivotal in managing intricate cases, as evidenced by their rising use during the COVID-19 pandemic.

3.3.2 Mobile health applications

Apps assisting in symptom evaluation and preliminary diagnosis can expedite the triage process. They empower patients to manage their health effectively and reduce the burden on ED resources.

3.4 Quality improvement tools

3.4.1 Root cause analysis (RCA)

Performing RCA following adverse events or near misses is vital. This method identifies deep-rooted issues in procedures or systems, paving the way for strategic improvements. It's a cornerstone of continuous quality improvement initiatives.

3.4.2 Simulation training

Conducting regular simulation drills for various emergency scenarios equips staff to handle a wide range of clinical situations. This training enhances response abilities, minimizes error rates, and fosters team coordination.

3.5 Communication and coordination tools

3.5.1 Centralized communication systems

Implementing systems like radio-frequency identification (RFID) for patient tracking and integrated communication platforms enables seamless coordination among various ED departments. This integration plays a crucial role in optimizing patient flow and resource utilization.

3.5.2 Standardized handoff protocols

Establishing consistent protocols for patient handoffs is key to minimizing information loss and ensuring continuity of care. These protocols are especially important during shift changes or when transferring patients between departments.

By embracing these methodologies and tools, the ED can markedly improve its risk management capabilities, leading to superior patient care and greater operational efficiency. These approaches not only address the immediate needs of patients but also contribute to building a more structured and dependable emergency care system.

Table 2 Comparative Table of Risk Management Methodologies and Tools in the emergency department provides a comprehensive overview, allowing readers to compare the various methodologies and tools discussed, highlighting their respective advantages, limitations, and ideal contexts for use. This comparative perspective aids in understanding the practical applications and potential impact of each tool and methodology within the dynamic environment of the ED.

Methodology/Tool	Advantages	Limitations	Ideal Use Context
Emergency severity index (ESI)	Enables quick patient triage based on severity.	Requires specific training for implementation.	High-volume EDs to prioritize critical cases.
Manchester Triage System	Standardizes patient assessment in urgent situations.	Less effective in extremely high patient volumes.	EDs with staff trained in the UK triage system.
Clinical Decision Tools (e.g., Ottawa Ankle Rules)	Reduces need for unnecessary diagnostic tests.	Specific to certain conditions; not applicable in all scenarios.	EDs for evaluating specific injuries, reducing X-ray burden.
Predictive Analytics (Data Analytics)	Predicts patient influx trends and resource needs.	Requires extensive and accurate historical data.	Large EDs with robust data collection systems.
Telemedicine	Improves access to specialists, reduces waiting times.	Depends on adequate technology and connectivity.	Remote EDs or those lacking onsite specialists.
Simulation Training	Enhances staff skills in realistic emergency scenarios.	Requires resources and time for simulations.	EDs looking to improve preparedness and response in critical situations.

ED: Emergency Department; ESI: Emergency Severity Index.

Table 2.
Comparative table of risk management methodologies and tools in the emergency department.

4. Challenges and limitations in implementing risk management tools and strategies

In the emergency department, effective implementation of risk management tools and strategies is crucial for enhancing patient care and operational efficiency. However, challenges such as resistance to change, technological limitations, training gaps, and regulatory and data security obstacles can complicate this process. In **Figure 2**, the process of implementing new technologies in the emergency department is outlined. It is essential to navigate through various stages: needs assessment, technology selection, planning, acquisition, staff training, implementation, and ongoing monitoring. This structured approach helps address the challenges and limitations mentioned.

One of the biggest challenges is resistance to change within the ED staff. The introduction of new methodologies and tools may be met with skepticism and reluctance, particularly from those accustomed to traditional practices. This resistance often stems from comfort with existing processes and doubts about the effectiveness of new methods. For example, at Massachusetts General Hospital, resistance to a new triage system was overcome through detailed training programs and feedback sessions that demonstrated tangible benefits of the system, such as reduced wait times and better patient classification. This change management approach emphasizes the importance of clearly communicating benefits and involving staff in the implementation process.

Technological limitations also present a significant barrier in some EDs, especially in rural or less developed areas. Limited access to high-speed internet, outdated hardware, or lack of system integration capabilities can hinder the effective

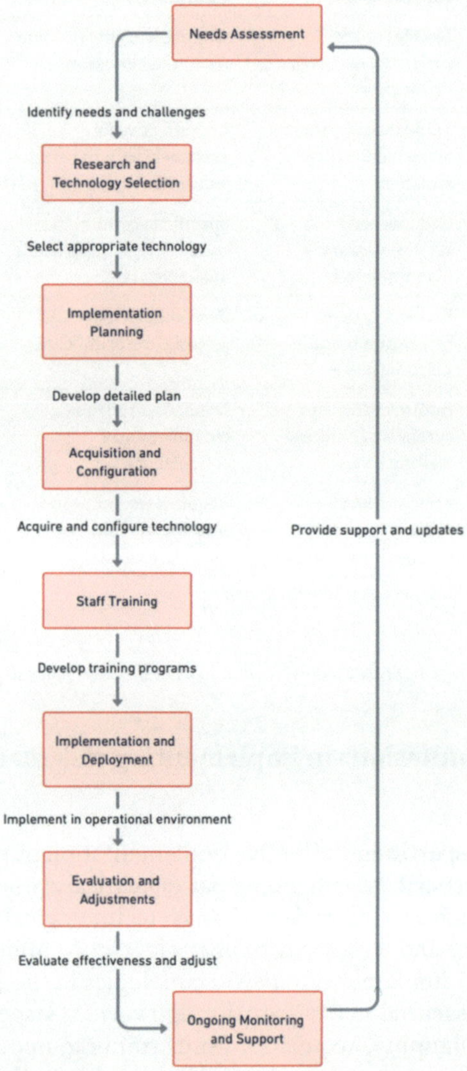

Figure 2.
Process of implementing new technologies in the Emergency Department.

implementation of tools like telemedicine or data analytics systems. Furthermore, staff may lack the necessary technical skills to fully utilize these tools, leading to underutilization or incorrect application. The experience of the University of Pittsburgh Medical Center illustrates how investment in advanced technological infrastructure and specific training in digital tools can significantly improve efficiency in the ED. They implemented an advanced electronic health record system and provided intensive training to staff, resulting in notable improvements in patient management and data accuracy.

Another area of focus is innovation in technology and processes. A prominent example is the use of telemedicine in the ED at Stanford Hospital, which has enabled rapid consultations with specialists and improved patient care in rural areas. This technological innovation has proven to be an effective tool for overcoming geographical and resource barriers.

Training and education gaps are crucial factors for the successful implementation of risk management tools. Without proper training, staff may not fully exploit the potential of these systems or could misuse them, leading to ineffective or suboptimal patient care. Continuous education and training are essential to ensure that ED staff are competent and confident in effectively utilizing these advanced tools.

Navigating the complex landscape of healthcare regulations and compliance requirements presents another challenge in integrating new risk management strategies. Ensuring that these tools and methodologies align with the latest legal and regulatory standards is critical but often complex, particularly with the rapidly changing nature of healthcare practices and technology.

With the growing reliance on digital tools and electronic health records, concerns about data security and patient privacy have become increasingly important. Ensuring the confidentiality and integrity of patient data while using advanced risk management tools is a major challenge that requires robust security protocols and constant vigilance.

To address these challenges, a comprehensive approach is necessary. This includes securing appropriate funding, fostering a culture receptive to innovation, providing thorough training and support, ensuring adequate technological infrastructure, and adhering to regulatory and data security standards. Addressing these issues is vital for the effective implementation of risk management tools and strategies, ultimately leading to improved patient outcomes and more efficient emergency care.

The growing incidence of overcrowding in EDs presents another crucial challenge. A study cited in the "Scandinavian Journal of Trauma, Resuscitation and Emergency Medicine" indicates that, over the past two decades, overcrowding in EDs has become an increasingly common global phenomenon. This overcrowding poses significant challenges as EDs must continue to provide care during periods of high demand and respond to both predictable changes (such as seasonal demand increases) and unexpected changes (such as unforeseen events and varying demand). Overcrowding hampers the ability of ED staff to provide timely, safe, and quality care, extending the time patients spend in the ED and threatening patient outcomes.

This overcrowding phenomenon underscores the importance of effective risk management in EDs, which should address not only the implementation of advanced tools and strategies but also consider how to optimally manage available resources during times of high demand. Challenges include not only technological and budgetary limitations but also the need for operational strategies that can quickly adapt to patient volume changes. Training staff in overcrowding management methods, along with implementing health information systems to improve communication and coordination, are key aspects of addressing this challenge. Furthermore, developing a culture that promotes adaptability and efficiency in managing patients during high-demand situations is essential for improving patient outcomes and maintaining the quality of care in the ED.

Finally, leadership plays a critical role in the successful implementation of new tools and strategies in the ED. Leaders must not only advocate for the adoption of innovations, but also ensure that staff are properly trained and supported during transition periods. The experience at Johns Hopkins Hospital's ED demonstrates how effective leadership, through the promotion of a culture of innovation and continuous learning, has led to significant improvements in risk management and patient outcomes.

5. Opportunities for enhancing risk Management in the emergency department

The dynamic and challenging environment presents numerous opportunities for enhancing risk management, improving patient care, and operational efficiency. These opportunities span from adopting advanced technologies to developing comprehensive training programs and embracing proactive change management practices.

The integration of emerging technologies like artificial intelligence (AI), virtual reality, and robotics offers transformative potential in the ED. AI systems, for instance, have been implemented in some hospitals to analyze patient data and predict potential deteriorations, thereby aiding in timely interventions. Virtual reality is increasingly being used for training purposes, providing realistic simulations that enhance the decision-making skills of ED staff. Robotics, though in its nascent stages, has begun to show potential in automating routine tasks, allowing staff to focus more on patient care.

Investing in advanced training and education programs is another key opportunity. These programs not only improve technical competencies but also foster adaptability and critical thinking. For example, Johns Hopkins Hospital has developed simulation-based training programs that prepare staff for complex and rapidly changing scenarios, enhancing their ability to manage various emergencies effectively. Additionally, workshops focusing on communication skills are becoming integral, as they are crucial in ensuring clear and effective interactions among staff and with patients.

Proactive change management practices are essential to leverage these opportunities effectively. Developing a culture that embraces change and innovation is critical. Effective leadership plays a vital role in this aspect, encouraging staff participation in decision-making processes and being open to experimenting with and learning from new approaches. A notable example is the Mayo Clinic, where leadership has consistently promoted a culture of innovation, leading to significant improvements in risk management and patient outcomes.

Collaborations and strategic partnerships have also proven beneficial. Partnerships between EDs and academic institutions, technology companies, and other healthcare organizations have led to knowledge exchange, resource access, and the development of innovative solutions in risk management. A case in point is the collaboration between Massachusetts General Hospital and a tech company to develop a predictive analytics tool that significantly improved patient triage and resource allocation in their ED.

Looking forward, the continuous improvement approach, where practices and processes are regularly reviewed and adjusted, will likely lead to significant advancements in the ED. Regular evaluations of implemented strategies and incorporating feedback from staff and patients are crucial for ongoing improvement. The future trends in risk management in the ED might include more personalized patient care approaches, enhanced use of data analytics for predictive modeling, and further integration of technology in everyday clinical practice.

The opportunities for enhancing risk management in the ED are abundant and varied. By leveraging technological innovations, focusing on advanced training and education, adopting proactive change management practices, establishing strategic collaborations, and committing to continuous improvement, EDs can significantly optimize patient care and operational efficiency. These opportunities not only benefit the patients but also empower the ED staff, contributing to a more dynamic, responsive, and rewarding work environment.

6. Conclusion

This chapter has thoroughly explored the critical aspects of risk management in the emergency department, covering everything from the identification of risk factors to the implementation of effective methodologies and tools, as well as the challenges and opportunities present in this dynamic environment. We have seen how technological innovation, advanced training, proactive change management practices, and strategic collaborations can significantly transform risk management in the ED. Looking forward, continuous adaptation and commitment to improvement are essential for evolving and consistently enhancing patient care and operational efficiency in EDs. This chapter provides a solid foundation for understanding and addressing these vital aspects, empowering healthcare professionals to effectively tackle challenges and seize opportunities in emergency care risk management.

Conflict of interest

The authors declare no conflict of interest.

Appendices and nomenclature

ED	emergency department
ECG	electrocardiogram
BP	blood pressure
ESI	emergency severity index
HR	heart rate
RR	respiratory rate
SpO_2	oxygen saturation
EHR	electronic health records
RCA	root cause analysis
RFID	radio-frequency identification

Author details

Rafael Suárez del Villar Carrero
Hospital HM Montepríncipe, Madrid, Spain

*Address all correspondence to: rsuarezdelvillar@hmhospitales.com

References

[1] Franklin A, Liu Y, Li Z, Nguyen V, Johnson TR, Robinson D, et al. Opportunistic decision making and complexity in emergency care. Journal of Biomedical Informatics. 2011;**44**(3):469-476. DOI: 10.1016/j.jbi.2011.04.001. Epub 2011 Apr 15

[2] Chiu H, Chung C. Risk management in emergency department. Hong Kong Journal of Emergency Medicine. 2000;**7**:96-103. DOI: 10.1177/102490790000700206

[3] Kim HI, Park S. Sepsis: Early recognition and optimized treatment. Tuberculosis and Respiratory Diseases (Seoul). 2019;**82**(1):6-14. DOI: 10.4046/trd.2018.0041 Epub 2018 Sep 28

[4] Tavirani MR, Beigvand HH. A review of various methods of management of risk in the field of emergency medicine. Open Access Macedonian Journal of Medical Sciences. 2019;**7**(23):4179-4187. DOI: 10.3889/oamjms.2019.616

[5] Fayfman M, Pasquel FJ, Umpierrez GE. Management of hyperglycemic crises: Diabetic ketoacidosis and hyperglycemic hyperosmolar state. The Medical Clinics of North America. 2017 May;**101**(3):587-606. DOI: 10.1016/j.mcna.2016.12.011

[6] Risk Management in emergency department. Omnia Health Insights. [Internet]. Available from: https://insights.omnia-health.com/medical-specialities/risk-management-emergency-department [Accessed: September 30, 2023]

[7] Canton LG. The emergency manager: Evolving roles and shifting paradigms. In: Emergency Management: Concept and Strategies for Effective Programs. John Wiley & Sons; 2006. pp. 63-83. DOI: 10.1002/9780470119761.ch3

[8] Lipe DN, Bourenane SS, Wattana MK, Gaeta S, Chaftari P, Cruz Carreras MT, et al. A modified emergency severity index level is associated with outcomes in cancer patients with COVID-19. The American Journal of Emergency Medicine. 2022;**54**:111-116. DOI: 10.1016/j.ajem.2022.02.002. Epub 2022 Feb 5

[9] Considine J, Fry M, Curtis K, et al. Systems for recognition and response to deteriorating emergency department patients: A scoping review. Scandinavian Journal of Trauma, Resuscitation and Emergency Medicine. 2021;**29**:69. DOI: 10.1186/s13049-021-00882-6

[10] Bessen T, Clark R, Shakib S, Hughes G. A multifaceted strategy for implementation of the Ottawa ankle rules in two emergency departments. BMJ. 2009;**339**:b3056. DOI: 10.1136/bmj.b3056

Chapter 3

Invasive Candidiasis: Risk Assessment for Predictor of Infection

Weny Rinawati

Abstract

Candidiasis is an infection caused by the *Candida* species. Invasive candidiasis is a severe and invasive form of infection, with manifestations that can be found in the blood (candidemia) or other organs (disseminated candidiasis). Early antifungal therapy is important for the management of invasive candidiasis and may reduce mortality. To date, the diagnosis of invasive candidiasis has been difficult and the criteria for empiric antifungal therapy have not been clearly defined. Risk assessment was developed as a clinical predictor to identify patients at risk of invasive candidiasis, provide appropriate and timely antifungal therapy, and avoid wasteful use of antifungal drugs. Risk assessments can be established based on the epidemiology of each health service or currently published risk assessments.

Keywords: *Candida* spp., invasive candidiasis, fungal infections, risk assessment, risk factor

1. Introduction

The location of infection is a common feature of fungal infections. These are classified as superficial, subcutaneous, and systemic which is also known as deep-seated. Several causes have been suggested for the sudden emergence of yeast species as causative agents of invasive infections. One of them is *Candida* species which is yeast fungi and normal flora. *Candida* species live in the mouth, throat, intestines, and vagina. However, colonization of *Candida* species can cause invasive candidiasis in at-risk patients. This infection can get into the blood and internal organs and also has the capability of spreading widely throughout the body. *Candida* infection in the blood is called candidemia, while in internal organs it is called disseminated candidiasis. Infected internal organs include the brain, heart, eyes, bones, or other parts of the body [1, 2].

Numerous impediments in the diagnosis of invasive candidiasis may delay the beginning of treatment. An atypical, dubious, and nonspecific early presenting symptoms driving the suspicion of a fungal infection, reduces the chance of making the proper clinical diagnosis [3]. The gold standard for the diagnosis of invasive candidiasis is cultured, but positive findings may be observed in cases of late infection. The drawbacks of culture are that it takes longer to receive examination results and cannot identify organ infections. Alternatively, it needs histopathology from normally sterile sites or organs, although necessitates invasive procedures and is often challenging. Since diagnosis of invasive candidiasis has many confinements, an approach to diagnosing invasive candidiasis can involve assessments that measure the risk of bacterial infections [3, 4]. In this chapter, we will discuss the definition, epidemiology, risk factors, pathogenesis, classification, diagnosis, management, and risk assessment of invasive candidiasis.

2. Invasive candidiasis

2.1 Definition

A fungal infection called candidiasis is brought on by this species. *Candida* species are 4–6 μm unicellular yeasts. Despite having thin cell walls, their structures include glycoproteins, β-glucan, chitin, and plasma membrane [5, 6]. The 1940s saw a rise in cases of candidiasis, which was correlated with the mass use of antibiotics, an increase in HIV infections, the use of therapeutic modalities for advanced life support, and specific surgical procedures like organ transplantation and prosthetic device implantation [7].

Almost all organs can become infected by *Candida* species. There are two different kinds of candidiasis invasive and superficial candidiasis. Superficial candidiasis refers to mild infections of the skin, nails, and mucous membranes, which the symptoms are paronychia and onychomycosis. Examples of skin symptoms of superficial candidiasis are perianal candidiasis and intertriginous candidiasis. Among the mucosal surfaces where superficial candidiasis might present include oral, perlece, candidiasis vaginitis and vulvovaginitis, candidiasis balanitis, and balanoptysis. A condition known as disseminated candidiasis occurs when *Candida* species enters the bloodstream and travels to several organs, resulting in symptoms including candidemia. Disseminated candidiasis can harm the heart, brain, eyes, bones, and other organs [1, 2].

2.2 Epidemiology

Seventy to ninety percent of fungal infections are caused by *Candida* species [4]. *Candida albicans* can be found in a variety of settings, including hospitals, food, animals, and inanimate items. Non-albicans species may live in environments with or without animals. In laboratories, contamination by *Candida* species occurs relatively seldom. In the past, substantial mistakes in patient care have resulted from a lack of comprehension of this idea. For example, positive cultures have been mistaken for skin or laboratory contamination. Typically found on the skin, in expectorated sputum, in the female vaginal canal, and in the urine of patients with indwelling Foley catheters, *Candida* species are human commensals. Healthcare workers are significantly more likely to be skin carriers [7].

It is nevertheless feasible for human-to-human transmission to happen even if the bulk of *Candida* infections are endogenous in origin. Examples are perinatal thrush, which can be contracted from a mother's vagina, and male circumcision infections from a spouse's *Candida* vaginitis-related balanitis. Not to mention, there's growing evidence that a hospital environment can be the source of a *Candida* infection. Molecular biology techniques significantly advance our knowledge of *Candida* epidemiology [7].

Of all the pathogens, *Candida* species is the most common, accounting for 17 percent of infections [3]. There has been a shift in the epidemiology of *Candida* species throughout the last two decades. Two-thirds of infections were formerly caused by *C. albicans*, which was the primary pathogen [4]. The sixth to tenth most common pathogen in Europe is a type of *Candida* [3]. Over the last few decades, non-albicans species have proliferated and are now responsible for up to 50% of infections; these species include *Candida glabrata, Candida krusei, Candida tropicalis*, and *Candida parapsilosis* [4].

Many variables, including individual risk factors, the prevalence of molecularly different *Candida* species specific to certain healthcare contexts, and local antifungal usage, frequently control the preponderance of non-albicans *Candida species* in most locations. *C. glabrata* is the second species that is most often seen in non-epidemic areas in the US and northwest Europe. Additionally, recipients of solid organ transplants and those over 60 are more likely to be members of this species. In comparison to *C. glabrata*, *C. parapsilosis* and/or *C. tropicalis* are significantly more prevalent in Southern Europe, India, and Pakistan. Out of all the five primary species of *Candida*, *C. krusei* is the least common. Data released in the previous 5 years indicate that *C. albicans* remains the most frequent species in South America. Notwithstanding country-specific variations, *C. parapsilosis* is the most prevalent non-albicans species [8].

A third of cases of candidemia were found in the intensive care unit (ICU) by Marchetti et al. [9]. ICUs had 5–10 times higher rates of candidiasis cases (2–6.7 per 1000 hospitalized patients) than standard wards. Five to 15% of patients have *Candida* species colonization when they are admitted to the intensive care unit (ICU). This percentage rises to 50–80% during treatment. Five to thirty percent of patients have invasive candidiasis five to 12 days after admission. Patients in the intensive care unit who stay longer than 7 days frequently develop multifocal colonization. The most common loci were the gastric (45.6%), oropharyngeal (34.3%), trachea (23.4%), perirectal area (21.2%), and urinary tract (18.7%). The relative risk of invasive candidiasis was significantly higher in patients with positive test findings for stool specimens (7.5% vs. 3.2%, $p = 0.019$) or urine (9.2% vs. 5.2%, $p = 0.032$) [4, 10].

While *Candida* species is the third and fourth most often isolated pathogen from blood cultures in the United States, accounting for 8–10% of bloodstream infections, it only causes 2–3% of bloodstream infections in Europe [3]. A previous research, Extended Prevalence of Infection in Intensive Care (EPIC) II (2011), found that 6.87 cases of candidemia occurred for every 1000 ICU patients [5]. The European ICU project (EUCANDICU, 2019) conducted a multinational, multicenter, retrospective examination in 23 ICUs across nine European nations as part of its first phase of research on intra-abdominal candidiasis and candidemia. The frequency of invasive candidiasis in ICUs in Europe was 7.07 episodes per 1000 ICU admissions, resulting in a crude 30-day mortality rate of 42% [11]. Invasive candidiasis has a mortality rate that ranges from 40 to 60% and can even reach 100% [3].

2.3 Risk factors

In the skin and mucosa, oropharynx, vagina, and large intestine, *Candida* species are found in their natural form. Neonates may colonize throughout the birthing process. Numerous risk factors for the development of invasive candidiasis are listed in **Table 1**. Pathogenic exposure to *Candida* species might occur during hospitalization or an ICU stay. Earlier colonization may have caused *Candida* organisms to translocate across the mucosa. Risk factors with a possible mechanism through

Possible cause of infection	Risk factor
Pathogenic exposure	Hospitalization or ICU
Translocation through the mucosa	Previous colonization
Immunosuppression	Premature and elderly
	Malnutrition
	Neutropenia (<500 cells/μL)
	Dialysis
	Malignancy
	HIV, AIDS
	Corticosteroids
	Chemotherapy
Facilitates fungal colonization Intravascular access	Broad spectrum antimicrobial
	Use of vascular catheter (CVC)
	Use of ventilators
	Use of TPN
	Major surgery or extensive burns
Genetics	Mutation in dectin-1, CARD 9, CD82, TLR1, or TLR2
	SNP at CD58, LCE4A-C1orf68, or TAGAP
	Vav protein

AIDS: Acquired Immunodeficiency Syndrome, CVC: central venous catheters, HIV: Human Immunodeficiency Virus, ICU: Intensive Care Unit, SNP: single nucleotide polymorphism, TLR: toll-like receptor, TPN: total parenteral nutrition.

Table 1.
Risk factors.

immunosuppression may result from prematurity and elderly (extreme age), malnutrition, neutropenia, HIV or AIDS, malignancy or other comorbidities, the use of corticosteroids, and chemotherapy. Meanwhile, the use of vascular catheters or ventilators, contaminated total parenteral nutrition, and major surgery or extensive burns can facilitate fungal colonization and direct vascular access [6].

Novel insights into immunity and the development of next-generation human antifungal therapies as components of tailored therapy have led to the introduction of a new chapter on risk factors. Mutations, single nucleotide polymorphisms (SNPs), and specific proteins like the Vav protein can all have an impact on invasive candidiasis [8].

2.4 Pathogenesis

Among the virulence factors that cause candidiasis include the capacity to switch (move from the yeast phase to the hyphal phase in infected organs), biofilm development, adherence by adhesins, and synthesis of extracellular hydrolytic enzymes including phospholipase and aspartyl protease [5, 7]. Although the yeast form is present on the surface of the epithelium and is necessary for the spread of systemic infections, the invasive form, hyphae, is necessary to infiltrate the epithelium and enter phagocytic cells [12, 13]. Extracellular hydrolytic enzymes play a critical role in overgrowth by facilitating tissue adhesion and allowing for host infiltration through penetration [13].

Mucous membranes and undamaged skin serve as the host's primary defensive mechanism against *Candida* species [7]. The immune response in the mucosa and epithelium enables the host to discriminate between invasive hyphal forms and yeast colonization [14]. Mitogen-activated protein kinase (MAPK) is triggered by hyphal growth, or it may be identified by looking for pathogen-associated molecular patterns (PAMP) of *Candida* species, such as β-glucan. After this realization, there is an inflammatory reaction. T-helper (Th17) differentiation requires macrophage IL-1 production, which is stimulated by hypopha development [13].

Candida species invasion might potentially exploit the host in cases of skin maceration or mucosal damage [7, 15]. In the process of colonizing, *Candida* species will accept host nutrients and attach to epithelium. *Candida* species use hydrolytic enzymes and hypha formation to cause surface infections and break down proteins in their hosts. In the event of immunological escape, *Candida* species have the ability to penetrate the tissue and adhere to the vascular endothelium [2, 15].

When endothelial adhesions form, the infection may penetrate organs and activate the coagulation system. *Candida* species are identified by leukocytes and can activate the complement system once they enter the bloodstream. Complement receptor 3 (CR3) and Fc gamma receptor (FcγR) are neutrophil receptors that recognize *Candida* species and establish signaling cascades that activate effector mechanisms like phagocytosis. Monocytes, as well as macrophages and dendritic cells found in numerous organs, play the role of mononuclear phagocytes. The cell identifies *Candida* species mostly through dectin-1 and induces IL-6 and tumor necrosis factor-α (TNF-α) release. *Candida* species are recognized by natural killer (NK) cells via pathogen recognition receptors (PRR), specifically NKp30. Perforin, which is secreted by NK cells, directly kills *candida*. Following that, NK cells produce granulocyte-macrophage colony-stimulating factor (GM-CSF) and interferon-γ (IFN-γ), both of which influence other immune cells [14].

2.5 Classification

The European Organization for Research and Treatment of Cancer/Invasive Fungal Infections Cooperative Group and the National Institute of Allergy and Infectious Diseases Mycoses Study Group (EORTC/MSG) introduced the revised definition of fungal disease. The definitions assigned 3 levels of probability to the diagnosis of invasive fungal infection, namely "proven," "probable," and "possible" invasive fungal infection. The category of proven invasive fungal disease can apply to any patient, regardless of whether the patient is immunocompromised, whereas the probable and possible categories are proposed for immunocompromised patients only [16].

The suggested definition of proven invasive candidiasis needed conclusive confirmation of the pathogen in a typically sterile location. It should include at least one of the following aspects [16]:

1. Histopathologic, cytopathologic, or direct microscopic examination of material obtained by needle aspiration or biopsy from a normally sterile site that shows budding cells consistent with *Candida* species (presence of pseudo-hyphae and/or true hyphae is highly suggestive of *Candida* species, but these structures are

not present in all *Candida* species and may be seen in other organisms, such as *Trichosporon* species, *Geotrichum* species, and *Magnusiomyces capitatus* [previously known as *Geotrichum capitatum*], as a result, validation using culture or PCR is required).

2. *Candida* species recovery by culture of a material acquired through a sterile technique (including a recently implanted [24 hours] drain) from a typically sterile location with a clinical or radiologic abnormality associated with an infectious disease process.

3. *Candida* species have been found in blood cultures.

The presence of at least one clinical criteria was used to define probable invasive candidiasis in the ICU (compatible ocular findings by fundoscopic examination, hepatosplenic lesions by computed tomography [CT], clinical or radiological (non-pulmonary) abnormalities consistent with an infectious disease process that are otherwise unexplained) plus at least 1 mycological criterion (positive serum 1,3-β-d-glucan in 2 consecutive samples, recovery of *Candida* in an intra-abdominal specimen obtained surgically or within 24 hours from external drainage), plus at least 1 of the following host factors [16].

The presence of at least one clinical criterion (fundoscopic evaluation of compatible ocular findings, computed tomography [CT] of hepatosplenic lesions, clinical or radiological (non-pulmonary) abnormalities associated with an infectious illness process but are otherwise inexplicable), at least one mycological criterion (positive serum 1,3-β-d-glucan levels in two consecutive tests; *Candida* recovery in an intra-abdominal specimen acquired surgically or within 24 hours of external drainage), and at least one of the following host variables was used to define probable invasive candidiasis in the ICU [16]:

1. Prednisone equivalent of 20 mg or higher per day glucocorticoid therapy

2. Neutrophil abnormalities, qualitative or quantitative (inherited neutrophil deficit, absolute neutrophil count 500 cells/μL)

3. Impairment of gut wall integrity (for example, recent abdominal surgery, chemotherapy, biliary tree abnormalities, repeated intestinal perforations, ascites, mucositis, acute pancreatitis, parenteral feeding)

4. Impaired cutaneous barriers to bloodstream infection (for example, the existence of a central vascular access device or hemodialysis)

5. *Candida* colonization is defined as the recovery of *Candida* species in cultures collected from two or more of the following sources: respiratory tract secretions, feces, skin, wound sites, urine, and drains left in place for 24 hours or longer

6. Hematopoietic stem cell transplantation (HSCT)

7. Solid-organ transplant (SOT)

2.6 Diagnosis

Clinical signs and symptoms, radiographic findings, culture, and histological abnormalities are all used to diagnose fungal infections. Clinical manifestation of invasive candidiasis is generally not specific and does not differ from another infection origin. It has a slow clinical course with vague signs and symptoms. Accurate diagnosis has lagged behind that caused by conventional pathogens such as bacteria and viruses. Proven invasive candidiasis usually requires confirmation with gold-standard methods [7, 17].

Although the culture-based method is the gold standard, it has limitations such as being insensitive and taking longer to acquire test findings [3, 17]. This approach has several drawbacks and may delay the initiation of proper treatment. Culture-based diagnostic approaches can only detect 50% of cases, and positive findings are possible in situations of late infection. The relevance of increased *Candida* recovery from places such as sputum, urine, feces, and skin is difficult to evaluate because the organisms can frequently be retrieved from these sites without producing infection [7].

Besides low sensitivity, taking specimens from sterile sites may be harmful to patients, therefore histological diagnosis is often challenging [3]. Commercial reagents for identifying and distinguishing *Candida* species thus develop for non-cultural diagnosis of invasive candidiasis. However, they are still not widely accessible at this time [18]. Despite the development of a considerable number of papers on the serologic diagnosis of disseminated candidiasis over at least three decades, disagreements over the use of various serodiagnostic methods persist [7]. Also, polymerase chain reaction (PCR) has lower reliability in the diagnosis of invasive candidiasis.

There is no single, fast, validated serodiagnostic test that is routinely used to diagnose invasive candidiasis at the moment. The β-glucan measurement is yielding a wealth of information. Because of false positives with this test, its greatest benefit may be in its substantial negative predictive value. Serial judgments may be useful in predicting therapeutic outcomes and serving as indicators of treatment effectiveness [7]. Radiological examination is also not specific for detecting certain infections. Halos or macronodules may not always be found, for example in patients with immunosuppression [3].

2.7 Treatment

The timing of antifungal medication in invasive candidiasis is critical to treatment effectiveness. The European Society of Clinical Microbiology and Infectious Disease (ESCMID) recommends four strategies for the management of invasive candidiasis, namely prophylactic, pre-emptive, empiric, and targeted therapy [4].

The goal of prophylactic antifungal therapy is to prevent the occurrence of invasive candidiasis in high-risk patients. For prophylactic therapy, most use fluconazole. Prophylactic use is rarely recommended for ICU patients. Pre-emptive therapy is antifungal therapy given from the start to patients with colonization and risk of candidiasis [19]. Pre-emptive therapy is given if there is microbiological evidence of invasive candidiasis, but clinical signs of fungal infection are absent or fit into the probable and possible categories, taking into account risk factors of invasive candidiasis in patients [4].

According to ESCMID recommendations, empiric therapy is given when persistent fever is present and there is a risk of fungal infection, but there is no microbiological evidence of invasive candidiasis, or only an increase is found during a risk assessment. Treatment was administered for a minimum of 14 additional days after the first negative culture result. De-escalation or switching to oral therapy is carried out after 10 days, taking into account the clinical picture [4].

Management can be adjusted to the therapeutic target if the culture results and sensitivity of *Candida* species are known. Patients are treated for a minimum of 14 days after the first negative culture result. De-escalation or switching to oral therapy can be done after 10 days, taking into account the clinical picture. Antifungals are given with therapy as recommended and within the antifungal spectrum [4].

3. Invasive candidiasis risk assessment

Invasive candidiasis risk assessment combines several risk factors into a scoring system to predict invasive candidiasis. This assessment has a good negative predictive value (NPV). It is useful for determining the risk of invasive candidiasis, and distinguishing patients with or without invasive candidiasis, which can address the possibility of antifungal overuse or underuse, increased healthcare costs, and the development of antifungal resistance [6].

3.1 Colonization index

The colonization index is the ratio of the number of colonizations in body areas other than blood, compared to the total number of cultures (**Table 2**). In the calculation, only the same *Candida* species strain is considered when calculating invasive candidiasis [19]. This risk assessment was made based on research by Pitett et al. [16]. Colonization was defined as finding *Candida* species in ≥3 specimens taken from ≥1 area on 2 consecutive screenings continuously [9]. Surveillance is carried out twice a week with specimens of oropharyngeal secretions, tracheal secretions, gastric fluid, perineum, feces, urine, surgical wounds, abdominal drains, and catheter insertion areas [20]. Data from 29 patients who met the inclusion criteria and were at high risk of candidiasis, there were 11 patients (38%) developed severe infections, 8 of them showed candidemia, while the other 18 patients showed colonization [19, 20]. All patients who developed candidiasis had colonization on average 6 days before candidiasis [17].

Risk factors that differentiate colonization from infection are the duration of previous antimicrobial therapy, disease severity according to the APACHE II, and *Candida* species. Based on logistic regression analysis, disease severity according to the APACHE II and *Candida* species colonization were independent factors for predicting invasive candidiasis. Colonization of *Candida* species precedes infection, with the same *Candida* species strain even though it is isolated from different areas of the body, and this pattern persists for up to 140 days [20, 21]. The colonization index of patients without infection and patients with infection, respectively, is 0.47 and 0.7, with a positive predictive value (PPV) of 66–100% [4, 20, 21].

The colonization index is corrected (Corrected Colonization Index, CCI), the ratio of the number of colonizations compared to the number of culture areas, multiplied by the ratio of the number of areas with fungal growth compared to positive areas, as seen in **Table 2**. CCI values <0.35 were found in colonization, and ≥0.4 in candidiasis. Sensitivity, specificity, NPV, and PPV are 100%. In multiple logistic regression

Index	Formulas	
Colonization index, CI	$CI = \frac{\text{Number of colonization areas}}{\text{Number of culture areas}}$	
	Colonization	0.47
	Invasive candidiasis	0.7
Corrected colonization index, CCI	$CCI = \frac{\text{Number of colonization areas}}{\text{Number of culture areas}} X \frac{\text{Number of areas with colony growth}}{\text{Total positive areas}}$	
	Colonization	<0.35
	Invasive candidiasis	≥0.4

Source: [20].

Table 2.
Description of colonization index.

analysis, independently only the APACHE II score and CCI score could predict the development of invasive candidiasis [20].

3.2 Paphitou rule

Paphitou rule includes criteria for hemodialysis, TPN use, diabetes mellitus, and use of broad-spectrum antimicrobials for ICU patients as shown in **Table 3**. The criteria were obtained based on a retrospective study by Paphitou et al. [22] of 327 patients who were treated in the surgical ICU for ≥4 days and had a risk of invasive candidiasis 11.0%. Patient data was collected from a week before entering the ICU until the third day of treatment in the ICU. Patients with combination diabetes mellitus, new-onset hemodialysis, TPN use, or broad-spectrum antimicrobial use had an invasive candidiasis rate of 16.6% versus 5.1% for patients who did not have these characteristics. Of the 52% of patients treated ≥4 days in the ICU, 78% of patients showed invasive candidiasis [22].

3.3 *Candida* score

Candida score is an inclusive risk assessment of four risk factors for invasive candidiasis, as in **Table 4**. These criteria are research-based Leon et al. [10] prospectively involved 1107 adult ICU patients treated between April 2006 and June 2007 in 36 ICUs in Spain, France, and Argentina. This study confirmed that the *Candida* score is a risk assessment to differentiate patients with severe sepsis or septic shock who would benefit

Variable
Hemodialysis
Use of TPN
Diabetes mellitus
Use of broad-spectrum antimicrobials

TPN: total parenteral nutrition.
Source: [22].

Table 3.
Paphitou rule.

Variable	Mark
Use of TPN	1
Operation	1
Multifocal *Candida* species	1
Severe sepsis	2

TPN: total parenteral nutrition.
Source: [10].

Table 4.
Candida score.

from early antifungals (*Candida* score > 3). Empirical antifungals are given if *Candida* score > 3, whereas if *Candida* score ≤3, no invasive candidiasis, and no antifungals [10].

The research of Leroy et al. [23] is a continuation of the research of Leon et al. [24], with subjects of 1669 adult ICU patients treated in 73 Spanish ICUs from May 1998 to January 1999. Four proven risk factors for invasive candidiasis were identified, namely total parenteral nutrition, surgery, multifocal *Candida* species colonization, and severe sepsis [23].

The four risk factors that constitute these variables are coded 1 if present, 0 if absent, and the *Candida* score is calculated according to the formula [23]:

Candida score = 0.908× (total parenteral nutrition) + 0.997 × (surgery) + 1.112 × (multifocal *Candida* species colonization) + 2.038 × (severe sepsis).

Based on receiver operating characteristics (ROC) and area under the ROC curve, a score of >2.5 can identify patients at risk of proven invasive candidiasis, with a sensitivity of 81%, specificity of 74%, NPV of 98%, and PPV of 16%, as seen in **Table 5**.

Li et al. [25] validated the revised *Candida* score model's clinical usefulness and comparative effectiveness, utilizing the Sepsis 3.0 criteria, in assessing critically sick patients over the conventional sepsis/severe sepsis model. The foundation for predicting the presence of invasive candidiasis should be Sepsis 3.0, given the clinical significance of organ failure in ICI.

3.4 Ostrosky-Zeichner rule

Ostrosky-Zeichner rule is a risk assessment based on a retrospective study by Ostrosky-Zeichner et al. [26] which was carried out on 2890 patients hospitalized

Variable	Value-based on	
	Leon et al. [24]	Leroy et al. [23]
Use of TPN	0.908	1
Operation	0.997	1
Multifocal *Candida* species	1112	1
Severe sepsis	2038	2
***Candida* score for invasive candidiasis**	>2.5	>3

TPN: total parenteral nutrition.
Source: [23, 24].

Table 5.
Candida score is based on research by Leon et al. [24] and Leroy et al. [23].

Major criteria	Minor criteria			
Systemic antimicrobial use (days 1 - 3) CVC use (days 1 - 3)	TPN use (days 1 - 3) Each dialysis (days 1-3) Any major surgery (days −7 - 0) Pancreatitis (day −7 - 0) Steroid use (days −7 – 3) Use of other immunosuppressives (days −7–0)			
Modification				
Use a ventilator for at least 48 hours				
Criteria	**Sensitivity**	**Specificity**	**PPV**	**NPV**
3 majors + >1 minor				
Without modification to major criteria	34	90	10	97
With modifications to the major criteria	50	83	10	97

CVC: central venous catheter, TPN: total parenteral nutrition.
Source: [22].

Table 6.
Ostrosky-Zeichner rule.

≥4 days at 9 hospitals in the United States and Brazil [25]. Initially, the major criteria for the Ostrosky-Zeichner rule were the use of systemic antimicrobials (days 1–3), and the use of a central venous catheter (days 1–3). Minor criteria are TPN use (days 1–3), any dialysis (days 1–3), any major surgery (days −7–0), pancreatitis (days −7–0), steroid use (days −7–3), or use of other immunosuppressives (days −7–0). These criteria can identify patients at high risk of invasive candidiasis. Invasive candidiasis among patients of the study subjects was 9.9%, with a relative risk of 4.36, sensitivity of 34%, specificity of 90%, PPV of 10%, and NPV of 97% (**Table 6**) [22, 27].

3.5 Nebraska medical center rules

Nebraska Medical Center rules is a risk assessment based on research by Hermsen et al. [28]. The criteria included in the Nebraska Medical Center rule risk assessment include those shown in **Table 7**. Hermsen et al. [28] conducted a retrospective

Variable	Score
Broad spectrum antimicrobial	1.5
Use of CVC	0.9
TPN use (days 1–3)	0.9
Use of steroids 7 days before entering the ICU until day 3	0.4
Abdominal surgery	0.9
Length of stay before being in the ICU x 0.039	
Nebraska Medical Center rules for invasive candidiasis	≥2.45

CVC: central venous catheter, TPN: total parenteral nutrition, ICU: Intensive Care Unit.
Source: [28].

Table 7.
Nebraska Medical Center rules.

matched case-control study from May 2003 to June 2008 to evaluate the sensitivity, specificity, PPV, and NPV of each criterion. These criteria include adults being treated in the ICU for ≥4 days, and invasive candidiasis matched with three controls based on age, gender, and date of ICU admission. If a score ≥2.45 is found, it is likely invasive candidiasis, with a sensitivity of 84.1%, specificity of 60.2%, PPV of 4.7%, and NPV of 99.4% [28].

3.6 Candidemia rule

The Candidemia rule is a risk assessment for candidemia in hospitalized patients with severe sepsis and septic shock, based on research conducted by Guillamet et al. [29]. The use of TPN, previous antimicrobial exposure, referral from an outside hospital or admission from a nursing home, mechanical ventilation, and the presence of a central venous catheter are independent predictors of candidemia, while the lung as a source of infection is protective, as seen in **Table 8**. Candidemia rule value <3 indicates no invasive candidiasis, while ≥3 indicates the presence of invasive candidiasis. These clinical prediction criteria for candidemia in hospitalized patients with severe sepsis and septic shock are better than previous risk assessments [29].

The study involved 2066 hospitalized patients with severe sepsis or septic shock who had positive blood cultures for *Candida* species. Severe sepsis and septic shock were proven by positive blood culture. Septic shock is characterized by the need for vasopressors (norepinephrine, vasopressin, dopamine, epinephrine, or phenylephrine). Candidemia is characterized by ≥1 positive blood culture result for *Candida* species, while bacteremia is when a positive blood culture is found for pathogenic bacteria. A central venous catheter is considered a risk factor if it was inserted a minimum of 48 hours before a positive blood culture. Immunosuppressive conditions included in the analysis included hematologic or solid organ malignancies, bone marrow transplantation, acquired immunodeficiency, long-term or high-dose corticosteroid administration, and chemotherapy and/or radiation therapy. This study also included criteria for a history of hospitalization in the previous 90 days, administration of antimicrobials, and bloodstream infections in the previous 30 days in the analysis. Antimicrobials that are suitable for treatment are preparations that

Variable	Score
Antimicrobials in the previous 30 days	2
CVC use >48 hours before positive blood culture	2
Use of TPN	2
Referral from nursing home	2
Referral from another hospital	1
Use of ventilators	1
Lungs as a source of severe sepsis or septic shock	−6
Candidemia rule for invasive candidiasis	≥3

CVC: central venous catheter, TPN: total parenteral nutrition.
Source: [29].

Table 8.
Candidemia rule.

have in vitro activity against the isolated organism and are administered at the correct dose during the first 24 hours after a positive blood culture result [29].

4. Conclusion

Invasive candidiasis, which includes both candidemia and deep-seated tissue candidiasis, is the most prevalent fungal illness among hospitalized patients. Early identification of invasive candidiasis is crucial in severely sick patients in particular. In individuals with invasive candidiasis at high risk, there is evidence of a correlation between delayed antifungal medication and higher mortality. For the purpose of starting preventative antifungal medication, many bedside technologies have been created for early invasive candidiasis detection. In addition to test diagnosis for invasive candidiasis, a risk assessment can be performed. Systemic candidiasis frequently occurs in the absence of candidemia, hence these two conditions must be combined. To foresee invasive candidiasis, it is suggested that a new risk prediction score be created using the logit model equation, which includes risk variables that take into account our own demography.

Author details

Weny Rinawati[1,2]

1 Doctoral Program of Medical Science, Faculty of Medicine, Universitas Airlangga, Surabaya, Indonesia

2 Department of Clinical Pathology, Laboratory and Blood Bank, National Brain Center Hospital Prof. Dr. dr. Mahar Mardjono, Jakarta, Indonesia

*Address all correspondence to: weny.rinawati-2022@fk.unair.ac.id; weny.rinawati@rspon.co.id

References

[1] Rinawati W, Kumalawati J, Bardosono S, Immanuel S, Sukartini N, Indrasari ND. Invasive candidiasis among high prevalence neurological patients. Journal of Infection in Developing Countries. 2022;**16**(5):871-880. DOI: 10.3855/jidc.15231

[2] Hermsen ED, Njoku J, Pfeifer R, Schooneveld TV. The Nebraska Medical Center Guidelines for Management of Invasive Candidiasis. Nebraska: The Nebraska Medical Center Clarkson and University Hospital; 2010

[3] Groth CM, Dodds-Ashley ES. Fungal infections in the ICU. In: Infection Critical Care. Lenexa: CCSAP; 2016. Available from: https://www.accp.com/docs/bookstore/ccsap/c2016b1_toc.pdf

[4] Hankovszky P, Társy D, Öveges N, Molnár Z. Invasive *Candida* infections in the ICU: Diagnosis and therapy. The Journal of Critical Care Medicine. 2015;**1**(4):129-139. DOI: 10.1515/jccm-2015-0025

[5] Kett DH, Azoulay E, Echeverria PM, Vincent JL. *Candida* bloodstream infections in intensive care units: Analysis of the extended prevalence of infection in intensive care unit study. Critical Care Medicine. 2011;**39**:665-670. DOI: 10.1097/CCM.0b013e318206c1ca

[6] Pfaller MA, Diekema DJ. Epidemiology of invasive mycoses in North America. Critical Reviews in Microbiology. 2010;**36**(1):1-53. DOI: 10.3109/10408410903241444

[7] Edwards JE. *Candida* species. In: Bennet JE, Dolin R, Blaser MJ, editors. Mandell, Dauglas, and Bennett's Principles and Practice of Infectious Disease. 8th ed. Philadelphia: Elsevier Saunders; 2015. pp. 2879-2894

[8] Riera FO, Caeiro JP, Angiolini SC, Vigezzi C, Rodriguez E, Icely PA, et al. Invasive candidiasis: Update and current challenges in the management of this mycosis in South America. Antibiotics (Basel). 2022;**11**(7):877. DOI: 10.3390/antibiotics11070877

[9] Marchetti O, Bille J, Fluckiger U, Eggimann P, Ruef C, Garbino J, et al. Fungal infection network of Switzerland. Epidemiology of candidemia in Swiss tertiary care hospitals: Secular trends, 1991-2000. Clinical Infectious Diseases. 2004;**38**(3):311-320. DOI: 10.1086/380637

[10] Leon C, Ruiz-Santana S, Saavedra P, Galvan B, Blanco A, Castro, et al. Usefulness of the "*Candida* score" for discriminating between *Candida* colonization and invasive candidiasis in non-neutropenic critically ill patients: A prospective multicenter study. Critical Care Medicine. 2009;**37**(5):1624-1633. DOI: 10.1097/CCM.0b013e31819daa14

[11] Bassetti M, Azoulay E, Kullberg BJ, Ruhnke M, Shoham S, Vazquez J, et al. EORTC/MSGERC definitions of invasive fungal diseases: Summary of activities of the intensive care unit working group. Clinical Infectious Diseases. 2021;**72**(Suppl. 2):S121-S127. DOI: 10.1093/cid/ciaa1751

[12] Lewis RE, Viale P, Kontoyiannis DP. The potential impact of antifungal drug resistance mechanisms on the host immune response to *Candida*. Virulence. 2012;**3**(4):368-376. DOI: 10.4161/viru.20746

[13] Singh G. Candidal infection: Epidemiology, pathogenesis and recent advances for diagnosis. Bulletin of Pharmaceutical and Medical Sciences. 2013;**1**(1):1-9

[14] Duggan S, Leonhardt I, Hunniger K, Kurzai O. Host response to *Candida albicans* bloodstream infection and sepsis. Virulence. 2015;**3**:1-11. DOI: 10.4161/21505594.2014.988096

[15] Cheng SC, Joosten LAB, Kullberg BJ, Netea MG. Interplay between *Candida albicans* and the mammalian innate host defense. Infection and Immunity. 2012;**80**(4):1304-1313. DOI: 10.1128/IAI.06146-11

[16] Donnelly JP, Chen SC, Kauffman CA, Steinbach WJ, Baddley JW, Verweij PE, et al. Revision and update of the consensus definitions of invasive fungal disease from the European Organization for Research and Treatment of cancer and the mycoses study group education and research consortium. Clinical Infectious Diseases. 2020;**71**(6):1367-1376. DOI: 10.1093/cid/ciz1008

[17] Barantsevich N, Barantsevich E. Diagnosis and treatment of invasive candidiasis. Antibiotics (Basel). 2022;**11**(6):718. DOI: 10.3390/antibiotics11060718

[18] Pittet D, Monod M, Suter PM, Frenk E, Auckenthaler R. *Candida* colonization and subsequent infections in critically ill surgical patients. Annals of Surgery. 1994;**220**(6):751-758. DOI: 10.1097/00000658-199412000-00008

[19] Kuwahara T, Shimono K, Kaneda S, Tamura T, Ichihara M, Nakashima Y. Growth of microorganisms in total parenteral nutrition solutions containing lipid. International Journal of Medical Sciences. 2010;**7**(3):101-109. DOI: 10.7150/ijms.7.101

[20] Eggimann P, Pittet D. *Candida* colonization index and subsequent infection in critically ill surgical patients: 20 years later. Intensive Care Medicine. 2014;**40**:1429-1448. DOI: 10.1007/s00134-014-3355-z

[21] Eggimann P, Pittet D. *Candida* colonization index in the management of critically iii patients. In: Vincent JL, editor. Yearbook of Intensive Care and Emergency Medicine. Yearbook of Intensive Care and Emergency Medicine. Vol. 2006. Berlin: Springer; 2006. DOI: 10.1007/3-540-33396-7_56

[22] Paphitou NI, Ostrosky-Zeichner L, Rex JH. Rules for identifying patients at increased risk for candidal infections in the surgical intensive care unit: Approach to developing practical criteria for systematic use in antifungal prophylaxis trials. Medical Mycology. 2005;**43**:235-243. DOI: 10.1080/13693780410001731619

[23] Leroy G, Lambiotte F, Thevenin D, Lemiere C, Parmentier E, Devos P, et al. Evaluation of "*Candida* score" in critically ill patients: A prospective, multicenter, observational, cohort study. Annals of Intens Care. 2011;**1**(50):1-7

[24] León C, Ruiz-Santana S, Saavedra P, Almirante B, Nolla-Salas J, Alvarez-Lerma F, et al. EPCAN Study Group. A bedside scoring system ("*Candida* score") for early antifungal treatment in nonneutropenic critically ill patients with Candida colonization. Critical Care Medicine. 2006;**34**(3):730-737. DOI: 10.1097/01.CCM.0000202208.37364.7D

[25] Li D, Zhang J, Han W, Bai G, Cheng W, Cui N. Evaluation of the updated "*Candida* score" with sepsis 3.0 criteria in critically ill patients. Annals of Translational Medicine. 2020;**8**(15):917. DOI: 10.21037/atm-20-995

[26] Ostrosky-Zeichner L, Sable C, Sobel J, dkk. Multicenter retrospective development and validation of a

clinical prediction rule for nosocomial invasive candidiasis in the intensive care setting. European Journal of Clinical Microbiology & Infectious Diseases. 2007;**26**:271-276. DOI: 10.1007/s10096-007-0270-z

[27] Ostrosky-Zeichner L, Pappas PG, Shoham S, Reboli A, Barron MA, Sims C, et al. Improvement of a clinical prediction rule for clinical trials on prophylaxis for invasive candidiasis in the intensive care unit. Mycoses. 2009;**54**:46-51. DOI: 10.1111/j.1439-0507.2009.01756.x

[28] Hermsen ED, Zapapas MK, Maiefski M, Rupp ME, Freifeld AG, Kalil AC. Validation and comparison of clinical prediction rules for invasive candidiasis in intensive care unit patients: A matched case-control study. Critical Care. 2011;**15**:R198. DOI: 10.1186/cc10366

[29] Guillamet CV, Vazquez R, Micek ST, Ursu O, Kollef M. Development and validation of a clinical prediction rule for candidemia in hospitalized patients with severe sepsis and septic shock. Journal of Critical Care. 2015;**30**:715-720. DOI: 10.1016/j.jcrc.2015.03.010

Chapter 4

Glycoconjugate Vaccine: An Effective Way to Combat Infectious Diseases and Cancers

Fatema Akter and Sanjeev Kumar

Abstract

Glycoconjugate is a molecule of carbohydrate covalently linked to another compound. In glycoconjugate vaccine, carbohydrate antigen is linked to another molecule, particularly a protein carrier. Vaccines targeting capsular polysaccharides can prevent bacterial infection. However, capsular polysaccharide alone is weak immunogenic as it produces a B cell immune response independent of T lymphocyte. To increase the immunogenicity, the capsular polysaccharide can be covalently linked to a protein carrier that converts carbohydrate antigen from T lymphocyte independent to T lymphocyte dependent antigen. Several carrier proteins such as tetanus toxoid (TT), diphtheria toxin (DT), the outer membrane protein complex (OMPC) of *N. meningitides* serogroup B, and *Haemophilus* protein D are currently used in licensed conjugate vaccines. The protein carrier in the glycoconjugate vaccine engages with T cell dependent immune response and the carbohydrate part engages with T cell independent immune response. The involvement of T cells in the immune response against the glycoconjugate vaccine helps in B cell proliferation and differentiation into memory B cell which is utmost important for long-term immunity. Carbohydrate structures decorated on the surface of pathogens and malignant cells can be considered as a key target in developing safe and effective vaccines to combat cancer, bacterial infections, viral infections.

Keywords: glycoconjugate vaccine, carrier protein, infectious diseases, malignant cells, T-cell dependent immune response

1. Introduction

Vaccines since its first use played a crucial role in the prevention, control and eradication (such as smallpox in humans and rinderpest in animals) of diseases. The mass immunization program against the diseases for which vaccines are available save countless live and economics losses in both humans and animals. The recent example include mass immunization of humans against SARS-CoV-2 (COVID-19) helped to reduce the mortality and hospitalization numbers. As per WHO data, current mass vaccination in children saved 2–3 million lives of children every year as result of that mortality in children of less than 5 years of age reduced from 93 deaths/1000 live births in year 1990 to 39 deaths/1000 live births in 2018. Vaccine is defined as a biological product that induces specific immune response against specific antigen and protects the individual against that disease on subsequent exposure to similar antigen [1]. An antigen may be anything such as a whole pathogen, small component of a pathogen, toxins produce by pathogen, etc. In the beginning of vaccine development, whole pathogen in the form of either live inactivated or killed was being used. With the advancement of medical science and biotechnological techniques, instead of using whole pathogen a small component of pathogens (subunit vaccine) that have both antigenicity and immunogenicity are being used for vaccine development. Moreover, many other platforms are being used for vaccine development such as DNA vaccines, recombinant protein vaccines, mRNA vaccine etc. The basic principle behind the protection given by vaccine is that vaccine induces the immune response against specific whole pathogen (either live, inactivated or killed) or small component of pathogen and immune system of body create a memory of this exposure in form of memory plasma cell, so that if individual gets exposure to same pathogen, it respond quickly without any delay, and clear the infection as soon as possible [2]. Whereas the naïve immune system starts developing antibodies after 7–10 days of its first exposure to antigen, called as primary response. But this primary antibody response consists of antibodies of IgM isotype that have low affinity for antigen. However, in primary response antibody titer is not enough and consists of IgM that is not sufficient to eliminate the infection completely. So, it is possible that animal may die due to delay immune response. The immune system requires more time approximately several days to few weeks to produce antibodies of either IgG, IgA or IgE isotypes that have the same antigen specificity but have high affinity to antigen [3]. Thus, mass immunization has been proved to be a very effective and economical way to prevent and control the diseases.

The word immunity is derived from the Latin word "*immunitas*" which is a legal status of Roman city-states that grants immunity to individuals from paying tributes to Rome or immunity from prosecution. In the first century, the Roman poet Lucan described the Psylli of North Africa as immune to the bites of venomous snakes in the Roman poem *De Bello Civile*. Similarly, the term diplomatic immunity indicates immunity to foreign government officials in the jurisdiction of the host country. Diplomatic immunity was first time guaranteed in 1709 by the British Parliament under the Diplomatic Privileges Act to foreign ambassadors after Count Andrey Matveyev, a Russian resident in London, was harassed verbally and physically by British bailiffs. Immunity is referred to as the ability of the immune system to protect the body from harmful pathogens and other substances/antigens. The fundamental function of the immune system is to differentiate between self and non-self antigens. And then, the non-self antigen is neutralized or eliminated by the immune system. The immune system is divided into two subtypes i.e. innate immune system and adaptive (acquired) immune system. The innate immune system consists of physical barriers (such as skin and mucous membranes), physiological barriers (such as temperature and pH), inflammatory mediators (such as complement, cytokines, interferon, acute phase protein, leukotrienes, etc.) and cellular components (polymorphonuclear cells, neutrophils, eosinophils, basophils, mast cells, monocytes and macrophages, dendritic cells). Using pattern recognition receptors (PRRs), innate immune cells may identify pathogens and tissue injury. Toll-like receptors (TLRs), which are found on the cell surface and in endosomes, were the first to be identified and are the best characterized. There are also more PRRs, including C-type lectin receptors on the cell surface and Retinoic acid-inducible gene-I (RIG-I) and Nucleotide oligomerization domain (NOD)-like receptors in the cytoplasm.

Innate immune system mediators are naturally present in a host since birth and are constitutive. However, innate immunity can also be induced, such as in the case of viral infection, virus-infected cells produce interferon that acts on non-infected cells and activates innate immunity against viral infection. The innate immune system is considered to be fast but rather nonspecific. The adaptive immune system consists of humoral and cell-mediated immune responses. The adaptive immune response is mediated by B lymphocytes and T lymphocytes. The humoral immune response is mediated by B lymphocytes and the cell-mediated response is mediated by T lymphocytes. In contrast to innate immunity, adaptive immunity has specificity in the recognition of foreign antigens by functional receptors residing on the cell surfaces of B lymphocyte (B cell receptor) and T lymphocyte (T cell receptor). An individual can acquire adaptive immunity either by direct contact of antigen with the immune system that leads to an immune response (either humoral or cell-mediated), called active immunity or by the acquisition of pre-formed antibodies and immune-reactive lymphocytes from another individual. Active adaptive immunity remains longer period (a few years) or sometimes gives lifelong immunity, whereas passive adaptive immunity remains for short period (a few weeks or months).

2. History of vaccines and immunization

Edward Jenner, an English Physician who discovered the smallpox vaccine using cow pox virus in year 1796, is considered as father of vaccine. Jenner collected matter from a cowpox sore on the hand of a milkmaid and inoculated into 8-year-old boy named James Phipps. Initially, James Phipps suffered from local reaction and ailing for several days but recovered soon and got lifelong immunity from smallpox. However, there are several evidence which show that the immunization practice has been started much before the Edward Jenner. In fifteenth century, people in different parts of world used to expose themselves intentionally to smallpox (by inhaling the crushed scab) to prevent the disease. In seventeenth century the Buddhist monks in China used to follow the practice of drinking snake venom to get immunity against the snake bite. Lady Mary Wortley Montagu brought smallpox inoculation to Europe in 1721. It is Benjamin Jesty, who in year 1774 tested his hypothesis that a cowpox virus when inoculated to human gives protection against smallpox. In May 1796, English Physician Edward Jenner expands on this discovery and inoculates 8-year-old James Phipps. Two months later, in July 1796, Jenner inoculates Phipps with matter from human smallpox sore in order to test Phipps' resistance. Phipps remains in perfect health and becomes the first human to be vaccinated against smallpox. The term 'vaccine' is later coined, taken from the Latin word for cow, vacca. It is very difficult to forget the achievements of Louis Pasteur in the development of vaccines. In 1872, despite enduring a stroke and the death of two of his daughters due to typhoid, Louis Pasteur creates the first laboratory-produced vaccine for fowl cholera in chickens. In 1885, Louis Pasteur was able to prevent the rabies successfully through 13 injections of post-exposure vaccination to 9 year old boy named Joseph Meister by using formalin inactivated rabies virus. Since then, many vaccines have been developed and many are in developing phase. On 30 January, 2020 the WHO Director General declares the outbreak of novel coronavirus 2019 (SARS-CoV-2) to be a Public Health Emergency of International Concern. On 11 March, WHO confirms that COVID-19 is a pandemic. Effective COVID-19 vaccines are developed, produced and distributed with unprecedented speed, some using new mRNA technology. In December 2020, just 1 year after the first case of COVID-19 was detected, the first COVID-19 vaccine doses are administered. The vaccine development usually take 10 to 15 years including clinical trials, however, it is the first time in history when COVID-19 vaccine was developed and administered to the patient in one year. The reason for this was that different phases of clinical trials overlap with each other.

3. Immunogenic vaccine antigen

Antigen is a substance (molecule) when introduced into the body induce a specific immune response (either humoral or cellular) or capable of binding with products of an immune response such as antibodies or lymphocytes [4]. Examples of antigens include proteins, carbohydrate, lipids, nucleic acid, toxins, any foreign particle (non-self-antigen) and sometimes bodies own tissue and cells (self-antigen). All immunogens are antigen but it is essential that all antigens are immunogens. For better understanding, few definitions are given below:

Immunogen: It is an antigen which is capable of inducing a specific immune response, called as immunogen. They can mobilize immune system and provoke immune response. *Incomplete antigen*: It is an antigen which can bind with specific antibody but unable to induce immune response by its own. These types of antigen need the help of other carrier molecule to behave as a complete antigen. They are also known as hapten. *Autoantigens*: There are some proteins such as lens proteins, sperm protein, myelin basic protein, thyroglobulin, kidney protein and some heart muscle protein that never participated in the process of immunogenic tolerance. Therefore, these proteins are recognized as foreign by T and B cells such that immune response is produced. Immunogenic tolerance to self-antigen *is acquired by clonal deletion or inactivation of developing lymphocytes*. *Allo-antigens*: These antigens are individual specific antigen present in one individuals but not in other. Examples of these antigens are blood group antigen and graft rejection. *Heterophilic antigen*: Antibodies produced by one antigen binds cross react with another antigen then such types of antigen are called as heterophilic or cross reacting antigen. For example, antibodies produced against *Rickettsia* bind with some *Proteus* species. Similarly, antibody produced against M protein of *Streptococcus pyogens* cross reacts with heart muscle protein of human. *Super antigens*: These types of antigens stimulate and cause proliferation of large fraction of T lymphocytes in non-specific manner. For example *Staphylococcus* enterotoxins, shock toxins, exfoliating toxin, pyrogenic exotoxins. *Antigenicity*: It is the ability of foreign molecule to combine specifically with products of immune response such as antibody or lymphocytes, is known as antigenicity. *Immunogenicity*: It is the ability of the foreign molecule (antigen) to induce immune response. Immunogenicity of an antigen depends upon four factors; how foreign an antigen compared to body, molecular size (antigen of large the molecular size is more immunogenic; >10,000 dalton), chemical composition (decreasing order of immunogenicity; Proteins > carbohydrate > Lipid > nucleic acids) generally do not act as antigen (immunogen) unless they are complexed with protein or carbohydrates) and their ability to be processed and presented on the surface of antigen presenting cells (APCs) such as dendritic cells, macrophage and B-cell. Some antigen needs the help of T cell for the production of antibodies. These types of antigens are called T cell dependent or thymus dependent antigen. Thymus dependent antigen induce both humoral as well as cell mediated immune response. On the other hand some antigen induces the antibody production without the help of T cell are called T cell independent or thymus independent antigen. Thymus independent antigen induces only humoral immune response. Antigens can be classified into exogenous antigen and endogenous antigen based on their origin. *Exogenous antigens* originate from outside and are foreign to host body. These antigens enter to the body either through inhalation, ingestion or injection. Whereas, *endogenous antigens* originate inside own body. These antigens are body's own tissues or cells or sub fragments or compounds or the antigenic products that are produced as a result of normal cell metabolism, or because of viral or intracellular bacterial infection. In vaccine production, mainly four types of antigens are used viz.; live inactivated whole pathogen, killed whole pathogen, toxoids and small component of whole pathogen.

4. Immune cells involved in immunization

First, it is very important to understand the different components of immune system. The immune system can be divided into two main subsystems; the innate immune system and acquired/adaptive immune system. The effective immune system is the result of interaction and co-ordination between innate and acquired immune system. There are four main differences between innate and acquired immune system. The first difference is that innate immune system is effective by birth, whereas, effective adaptive immune system develop with time as body acquires natural infections. The second difference is that innate immune system act in non-specific manner, whereas, adaptive immune system act in specific manner for specific pathogen/antigen. In literal meaning, innate immune system uses same weapon to all pathogen, whereas acquired immune system uses different weapons to different pathogen. The third difference is that innate immune system keeps no memory of antigen exposure, whereas adaptive immune system keeps memory of antigen exposure. The fourth difference is that the innate immune system is very fast (takes minutes to hours to respond) compared to adaptive immune response (takes few days to weeks to respond). However, the adaptive immune system has memory which means that the adaptive immune system will respond more rapidly to that particular pathogen with each successive exposure. The innate immune system includes anatomic barriers such as intact skin and mucous membranes, physiologic barriers as the normal body temperature, fever, gastric acidity, lysozyme, interferon, and collectins. The complement pathways are also a part of the defensive measures of the innate immune system. The inflammatory response is another essential part of the innate immune response. The inflammatory response allows products of immune system into area of infection or damage. The adaptive immune response is composed of the B cells/antibodies and T cells. Natural killer cells are also from the lymphocyte lineage like B cells and T cells; however, natural killer cells are only involved in innate immune responses. For an immune response to be effective, both the innate and adaptive immune systems must function. B cells that make antibodies (humoral immunity) and T cells (cellular immunity) are the mediators of the adaptive immune response. Additionally, in order for immunization to be effective, effector cells and memory cells need to be produced in order to cause long-term stimulation of the adaptive system's humoral and cell-mediated arms. The body must first recognize the threat, whether it be a pathogenic agent or an immunization, as with any challenge to the immune system. Although B cells may also carry out this initial detection, the innate immune system typically handles this task. When the immune system detects antigen epitopes, the detection process starts. Small areas on antigens called epitopes mimic immune recognition. The innate immune system's various components will then react to this threat. These innate immune system elements will opsonize or bind to the pathogen, assisting antigen-presenting cells like macrophages or monocytes in engulfing it. The pathogenic agent's antigens will then be processed by these antigen-presenting cell(s), and they will be added to the surface of the antigen-presenting cell along with the MHC protein. If the antigen is viral or endogenous, the MHC-I protein will bind to it and the antigen-presenting cell will present it to a CD8+ T cell, which is likely to result in cell-mediated immunity. If the antigen is bacterial or parasitic or other exogenous antigen, MHC-II protein will bind to it and the antigen will be presented by the antigen-presenting cell to a CD4+ T cell, likely inducing antibody-mediated immunity. The majority of current vaccines are thought to confer protection primarily through the induction of antibodies, with the exception of BCG (which is thought to induce T cell responses that prevent severe disease and innate immune responses that may inhibit infection). There is a number of evidence to support the idea that different types of functional antibodies play a crucial role in vaccine-induced immunity, and it primarily comes from three different places: studies of passive immunity, immunological data, and immunodeficiency conditions.

5. Vaccine types

Vaccines are generally classified as live or non-live/ inactivated. Live vaccines contain those attenuated replicating strains of the relevant pathogenic organism. Non-live/inactivated vaccines contain killed whole organisms. Several other platforms, such as viral vectors, nucleic acid-based RNA and DNA vaccines, and virus-like particles, have been created over the past few decades in addition to the "traditional" live and non-live vaccines. It's crucial to understand the difference between live and non-live vaccines. The live vaccines may have the potential to replicate uncontrollably in immune-compromised individuals resulting in some limitations on their use. Non-live vaccines, on the other hand, pose no risk to immune-compromised individuals. Example of live vaccines include measles, mumps, rubella and rotavirus vaccines, oral polio vaccine, BCG vaccine, and live attenuated influenza vaccine. Inactivated vaccines, on the other hand, do not always elicit as strong or long-lasting immune responses as live attenuated vaccines. Examples of inactivated vaccines include inactivated Polio vaccine, Hepatitis A vaccine, etc. In subunit vaccines, which contain no whole bacteria or viruses. Instead, these vaccines often include one or more particular pathogen-surface antigens. Subunit vaccinations provide an advantage over complete pathogen vaccines in that the immune response can concentrate on identifying a limited set of antigen targets. Subunit vaccinations frequently fail to elicit the same robust or durable immune response as live attenuated vaccines. Initially, they often call for repeated dosages, followed by booster dosage the following year. Subunit vaccinations frequently have adjuvants added. Adjuvants are the substances that support and prolong the immunological response to the vaccine. Aluminum salts (alum) have been extensively used as adjuvants for more than 80 years (HPV). The oil-in-water emulsion MF59, AS01 and AS04, are examples of novel adjuvants. As a result, with these kinds of immunizations, typical local reaction could be more obvious and frequent. In recombinant vaccines, a tiny fragment of DNA from the virus or bacterium that we want to protect ourselves from is obtained and introduced into the production cells. For instance, a portion of the DNA from the hepatitis B virus is introduced into the DNA of yeast cells to create the hepatitis B vaccine. Once one of the hepatitis B virus's surface proteins is produced by these yeast cells, it is purified and employed as the vaccine's active component. Recombinant vaccine examples include MenB vaccine, HPV vaccine, and hepatitis B vaccine. This has proteins from the outer layer of meningococcal bacteria. The recombinant method was used to create three of the proteins. Toxins generated by bacteria are inactivated in toxoid vaccinations using formalin or heat to lessen pathogenicity and are used as vaccine. These toxins can elicit an immune response despite being inactive and safe. Diphtheria, tetanus, and pertussis (whooping cough) vaccines are a few examples of toxoid vaccines. Toxoid and surface-derived proteins from the pertussis bacteria are both included in the pertussis vaccine. The vaccination is frequently described as "acellular." In virus-like particles (VLPs), viral genetic material is absent which are entities that closely resemble viruses but are not infectious. They exist naturally or are created through individual expression of viral structural proteins, after which they self-assemble into forms that resemble viruses. In other circumstances, the viral structural proteins themselves serve as VLP vaccination antigens. As an alternative, VLPs can be created to display antigens from many diseases on their surface or to do so simultaneously. Due to the fact that each VLP includes numerous copies of an antigen on its surface, it can more efficiently elicit an immune response than a single copy. Outer member vesicles (OMV) vaccines are a more recent development in vaccine technology. Membrane vesicles (OMVs), which contain many of the antigens on the cell membrane, are naturally produced by bacteria. To create vaccines, these OMVs can be extracted from bacteria. The OMVs can also be altered to keep the antigens that are good at triggering an immune response while removing the harmful antigens. OMVs also function as adjuvants by nature. The MenB vaccine is authorized to use this technology. In contrast to conventional vaccines, nucleic acid vaccines do not provide the protein antigen, thus they operate differently. Instead, they impart the genetic code for the antigen to body cells, which then produce the antigen and trigger an immune response. Nucleic acid vaccines are quick and easy to develop and provide significant promise for the development of vaccines in the future. RNA vaccines and DNA vaccines are the two categories into which nucleic acid vaccines fall. In an RNA vaccination, messenger RNA is enclosed in a lipid membrane. When the mRNA first enters the body, its fatty layer protects it. However, it also facilitates entry into cells by joining with the cell membrane. The mRNA is translated into the antigen protein by internal cell machinery once it has entered the cell. Although this mRNA only persists for a few days on average, enough antigen is produced during that period to elicit an immunological response. The body then naturally breaks it down and eliminates it. RNA vaccines are unable to interact with the genetic code of humans (DNA). Currently, the UK has approved the use of two RNA vaccines for emergency situations. The COVID-19 vaccines from Moderna and Pfizer BioNTech are both made of RNA. DNA vaccines do not need the same initial protection because DNA is more stable than mRNA. DNA vaccinations are frequently given combined with a process known as electroporation. This enables the body's cells to absorb the DNA vaccination by using low-frequency electrical waves. Before DNA can be translated into protein antigens that trigger an immune response, it first needs to be transcribed into mRNA in the cell nucleus. Although there are several DNA vaccines being developed, there are currently no licensed DNA vaccines available for commercial use. A more recent development in vaccine development is the use of viruses to carry the genetic code of the target antigens of the vaccine to body cells, where the cells can then create protein antigens to elicit an immune response. Viral vectored vaccines can be produced rapidly and easily on a wide scale since they can be generated in cell lines. When compared to nucleic acid vaccines and many subunit vaccines, viral vectored vaccines are typically produced at a significant cost savings. There are two types of viral vectored vaccines, depending on whether a replicating or non-replicating vector was utilized. When utilized as a platform for vaccine delivery, replicating viral vector vaccines retain the capacity to produce new viral particles in addition to delivering the vaccine antigen. This replicating virus, like live attenuated whole pathogen vaccines, has the intrinsic benefit over non-replicating vaccines in that it may supply a continuous stream of vaccine antigen over an extended period of time, which is likely to result in a higher immune response. Protection may be provided by a single vaccination. Replicating viral vectors are often chosen so that the viruses are attenuated or harmless, preventing disease while they are infecting the host. Despite this, there is a higher likelihood of moderate adverse reactions with these vaccines since viral replication is still occurring. Recombinant vesicular stomatitis virus is used in the Ebola vaccine Ervebo (rVSV-ZEBOV). Over 90,000 people were protected by this vaccination during several Ebola outbreaks in Europe in 2019 after it received approval. The vaccine has mostly been employed in "ring vaccination," which immunizes a person's close contacts in order to stop the virus from spreading. When a vaccine uses a non-replicating viral vector, the vector nevertheless has the capacity to produce new virus particles while delivering the vaccine antigen to the cell. This is due to the deletion of essential viral genes required for viral replication. The vaccine cannot induce disease and adverse events linked to viral vector replication are also decreased. But only while the initial vaccine is still present in infected cells, vaccine antigen can be generated (a few days). Accordingly, booster doses are probably

S. N.	Platform	Example
1	Live attenuated whole pathogen	Measles, mumps, rubella, yellow fever, influenza, oral polio, typhoid, Japanese encephalitis, rotavirus, BCG, varicella zoster
2	Killed whole pathogen	Whole-cell pertussis, polio, influenza, Japanese encephalitis, hepatitis A, rabies
3	Toxoid	Tetanus, diphtheria
4	Subunit vaccine	Pertussis, influenza, hepatitis B, meningococcal, pneumococcal, typhoid, hepatitis A, SARS-CoV-2
5	Virus like particle (VLP)	Human papillomavirus, hepatitis B virus
6	Protein-polysaccharide conjugate	*Haemophilus influenzae* type B, pneumococcal, meningococcal, typhoid
7	Viral vectored	Ebola, SARS-CoV-2
8	Outer membrane vessicle	Group B meningococcal
9	RNA vaccine (mRNA)	SARS-CoV-2
10	DNA vaccine	SARS-CoV-2, West Nile Virus in horses, Melanoma vaccine for dogs
11	Bacterial vectored	Experimental
12	Antigen presenting cells	Experimental

Table 1.
Different platforms used for vaccine development.

necessary because the immune response is typically less than with viral vectors that can replicate themselves. A non-replicating viral vector with the name of ChAdOx1 is also used in the Oxford-AstraZeneca COVID-19 vaccine, which was authorized for use in emergency situations. The conjugate vaccine type is another challenging area with a numbers of successful vaccines available commercially. In conjugate vaccine, a hapten (polysaccharide or other molecules) is coupled to a carrier molecule. The polysaccharide is joined to diphtheria or tetanus toxoid protein (carrier) in the majority of conjugate vaccines which are specifically termed as glycoconjugate vaccine. These carrier molecules merely make the hapten more visible to the immune system. These proteins are relatively simple for the immune system to recognize, which contributes to a greater immunological reaction to the polysaccharide. MenC vaccine, Pneumococcal (PCV) vaccine, MenACWY vaccine, and Typhoid Conjugate Vaccine (TCV) are a few examples of glycoconjugate vaccines. Glycoconjugate vaccines are discussed further in detail. List of various platforms for vaccine development included in the **Table 1**.

6. Glycoconjugate vaccine

Glycoconjugate vaccines are formed when a polysaccharide (mostly bacterial) is covalently linked with a protein providing epitopes for T lymphocyte which are required in the germinal centers for the affinity maturation of polysaccharide-specific B lymphocytes. Research has been shown that the bacterial conjugate vaccines can be used in all the age grouped including infants, adolescents, and the elderly, and are found to be among the safest and most successful vaccines developed during the last 40 years [5]. The theory of conjugate vaccine (glycans covalently linked to immunogenic proteins) was studied for the first time by Avery in the year 1931, and was introduced in the area of Antibacterial Vaccine in 90s [6]. There is a positive benefit of the glycoconjugate vaccines which when taken up by antigen-presenting cells, the conjugate molecule gets digested and the covalently-linked fragments of both polysaccharides and proteins are able to bind with the major histocompatibility complex II (MHC-II). This is then presented to T lymphocytes which in turn results to isotype switching from IgM to IgG and also induce B cell differentiation into memory cells, together act as a good vaccine. Tumor markers such as gangliosides, sialic acid-containing glycosphingolipids with extracellular polysaccharide head groups are expressed at high levels on the surface of cancer cells which are readily available to interact with the immune cells in turn acts as an antigen for cancer cells and becoming a potential cancer vaccine target. Though they have been proved to be a poor antigen but when synthetic antigen of gangliosides linked to polyamidoamine scaffolds to induce responses in γδ T lymphocyte receptor and CD8+ phenotypes was found to be therapeutic. For a glycoconjugate vaccine to be produced, each parts are prepared individually followed by conjugation of both the components into one molecule where only the polysaccharide part remains unique for each given vaccine. Traditionally a small group of proteins is used after inactivation of toxins that is toxoids. Toxins produced by some pathogenic cells or bacteria (can be used as bio-factories), are inactivated with formaldehyde or any other inactivating agents shown strong antigenicity and safe, for example tetanus toxoid (TT) has been used since 1924 till today. There is also possibility to use relatively nontoxic mutants including Cross Reactive Material 197 (CRM197) than the diphtheria toxoid (DT) [7]. The mechanism of how glycoconjugate vaccine works are briefed in the **Figure 1**.

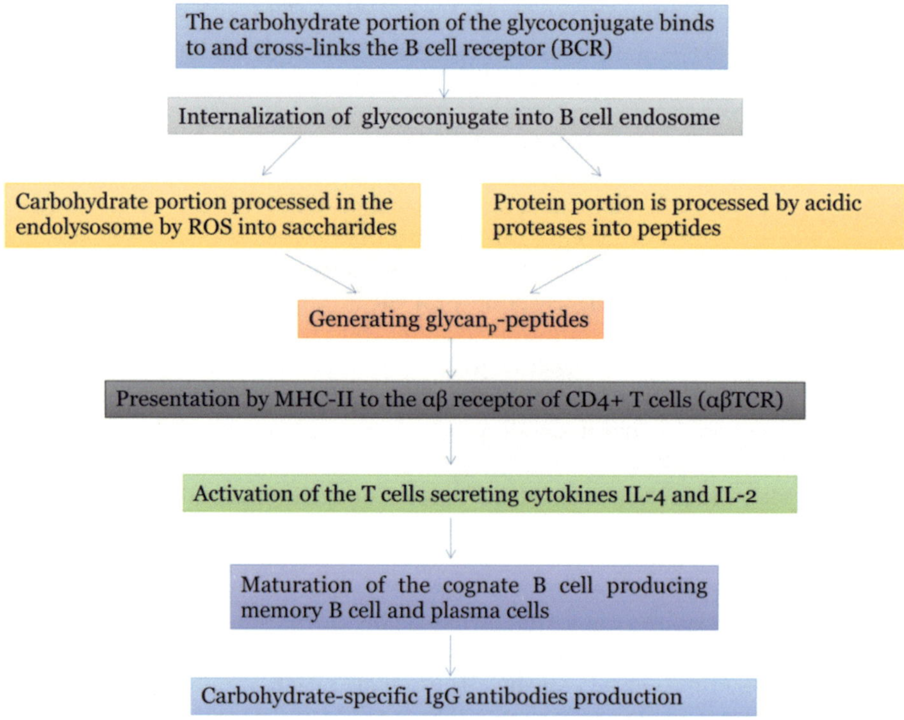

Figure 1.
Proposed mechanism of action of glycoconjugate vaccine to induce immune response.

7. Glycoconjugate vaccine production

There are three pathways for glycoconjugate vaccine production including:

1. Coupling of monofunctional oligosaccharides (after depolymerisation of the parent polysaccharide) or bifunctional oligosaccharides at low coupling efficiency, and either through direct attachment to the carrier protein or indirect attachment through a linker.

2. Activation of higher molecular weight polysaccharides without depolymerisation and conjugation through non-specific chemistry to multiple carrier proteins to give a very high molecular weight complex of >1 MDa size.

3. Reduced mass polysaccharides with multiple activations coupled to LPS-depleted outer membrane protein (OMP) vesicles.

Though the most of the protein carriers are related to toxins, there are also a various known proteins which can be used as carrier including keyhole limpet hemocyanin is being used as a carrier for glycoconjugate vaccines against *Candida albicans* [8]. Bovine serum albumin (BSA) which is a well characterized protein is also used as carrier for glycoconjugate vaccine against *Aspergillus fumigates* [9]. The polysaccharide part on the other hand is produced enzymatically rendering polydispersity which again depends on the kinetics, thermodynamics, and relative proportions of subunits and enzymes during the polysaccharide production. It is also possible to synthesize the small fragments *in vitro*. Although advances have been made for synthesis and fractionation where polysaccharides are near-monodisperse. After both the components are ready, then the step includes is the covalent linking. As the surface of each molecule possesses a number of functional group with a potential to generate a covalent link under the right conditions. One way to reduce the polydispersity is to target the formation of specific bonds which has been described by Adamo et al. [10]. As a vaccine to be effective, the first and one of the important trait is the stability of the each components and their covalent linker, although the most important component which needs to be stable is the polysaccharide so that it is able to mimic accurately the structure of the target antigen, whereas the protein only needs to be recognized as non-self by the antigen presenting cell (APC). To learn about the integrity of the conjugated vaccines, there are physicochemical methods including high field nuclear magnetic resonance (NMR) spectroscopy [11], analytical ultracentrifugation (AUC) [12], which have been proven to be important in determining their molecular integrity.

8. Carriers of glycoconjugate vaccine

The most widely used carriers are protein based. The commonly used carrier proteins are TT (tetanus toxoid), DT (diphtheria toxoid), OMPC (outer membrane protein complex of *Neisseria meningitides* serogroup B), *Haemophilus* protein D, and CRM197 (Cross Reactive Material 197, mutant of DT). Studies showed that the stability of these carriers have negative effect when stored at −20°C, while they remain stable at 2–8°C storage temperature [7, 13]. A study performed by Togashi et al. [14] to compare the TT and CRM197 carriers for PRP (Polyribosyl Ribitol Phosphate) showed no significant differences, but it was observed that the CRM197 conjugate has higher local reaction. In another study by Akeda et al. [15] showed that the CRM197 has higher bactericidal action in comparison with TT. When the tri-component synapse of processed antigen; MHC- II; and T cell receptor is formed, the T helper cell provides stimulatory and cytokine-mediated signals to B-cells to release high affinity immunoglobulin G (IgG) and also memory B cells which gives a long-term immune response [6]. The other type of carriers which is also used for glycoconjugate vaccines is oligodeoxynucleotide and lipid carriers which targets TLRs (Toll-like receptors). Research is going on to find out the effectiveness of this carrier. The CpG-ODN (cytosine-phosphate-guanosine-oligodeoxynucleotides) has been used as an external adjuvant in a polysaccharide-protein conjugated vaccine to increase antibacterial immune response against *S. pneumoniae* polysaccharide types 19F and 6B [16]. The co-administration of CpG with *H. influenzae* type b (Hib) polysaccharide conjugate vaccine on mice model showed to increase the neutralizing antibody titer against both the polysaccharide and the Hib [17]. The *N. meningitidis* monophosphorylated lipid A (MPLA) conjugated with CPS of *N. meningitides* serotype C was evaluated in a mice model to learn the immunogenicity of MPLA conjugate. The MPLA glycoconjugates which were inoculated as liposomal formulations showed greater immunity as compared to the traditional protein glycoconjugates including adjuvant [18]. On the other side, when the tetrasaccharide of Mycobacterial LAM (lipoarabinomannan) was conjugated to the primary position of glucosamine residue of MPLA showed a robust IgG response in mice, indicating the structure of the linker and the conjugation site of the carbohydrate antigen epitope on MLPA has a key role to play in the immune response [6, 19]. The third type of carrier is nanoglycoconjugate where glycol-liposomes has been considered as a good alternative of covalent conjugation of protein and bacterial saccharide antigen [20]. The work of Hassane et al. [21] is a good example of use of nanoglycoconjugate carrier for *Shigella flexneri* vaccine formulation. In their studies, they have used synthetic liposomes with two sets of *S. flexneri* 2a synthetic pentasaccharides which are B cell epitopes mimicking the O antigen of *S. flexneri* and universal T_H epitope from hemagglutinin (HA) 307–319 of Influenza virus. It showed effective antibody response against the native lipopolysaccharide *in vivo.*

9. Advances in glycoconjugate vaccine

Recently there are glycoconjugate vaccines which are successfully licensed worldwide against *H. influenzae*; meningococcus serogroups A, C, and ACWY; pneumococcus serotypes 10 to 13; and *Salmonella typhi*. The list of licensed glycoconjugate vaccines are mentioned in the **Table 2**. Altogether these vaccines has made a history by reducing the global infant mortality and morbidity by eliminating some of these diseases including, meningococcus C eliminated from the United Kingdom after a huge vaccination campaign in 1999, and outbreaks of meningococcus A has also been eliminated from the African meningitis belt, resulting in great reduction in the global occurrence of bacterial meningitis and pneumonia [5]. Borja-Tabora et al. [22] and Holme et al. [23] experimented using a meningococcal vaccine (Men) with the serotypes A, C, W and Y polysaccharides which were either linked with TT (tetanus toxoid) as a glycoconjugate or as a polysaccharide only vaccine. In both the experiments, they have found higher and persistent antibody response where the patients were vaccinated with conjugate rather than polysaccharide only vaccine. Ramasamy et al. [24] in their experiment using conjugated and polysaccharide vaccines, observed differences in the antibody titer. They have observed that the polysaccharide vaccine has higher efficacy against meningococcus serotype C strains, whereas the conjugated vaccine showed higher efficacy against serotype W. They have concluded that these differences may be because of the lower titer

Vaccine (manufacturer)	Licensed in (year)	Target organism	Carrier protein
Pedvax-Hib (Merck Sharp & Dohme Corp, USA)	1990	*Haemophilus influenzae*	OMP
ActHib (Sanofi Pasteur SA, France)	1993	*Haemophilus influenzae*	TT
Menactra (Sanofi Pasteur Inc., USA)	2005	*Neisseria meningitidis*	DT
Hiberix (GSK, Belgium)	2009	*Haemophilus influenzae*	TT
Menveo (GSK, Italy)	2010	*Neisseria meningitidis*	CRM197
Prevnar 13 (Pfizer, USA)	2010	*Streptococcus pneumoniae*	CRM197
Typbar-TVC (Bharat Biotech Ltd., India)	2019	*Salmonella typhi*	TT
MenQuadfi (Sanofi Pasteur Inc., USA)	2020	*Neisseria meningitidis*	TT

Table 2.
Licensed glycoconjugate vaccines.

of polysaccharide C which was conjugated with the CRM197 protein. Rothstein et al. [25] performed experiment using various combinations of conjugated and unconjugated vaccines against *Haemophilus influenza* type b on 7–15 month old infants with three time inoculations. They have observed that there was similar mean antibody titer when used all the three inoculations with conjugated vaccine, and when only the last inoculation was replaced with pure polysaccharides. On the other hand, there was decreased antibody titer when two inoculations were replaced with polysaccharide. These results tell us that the glycoconjugate vaccines show good antibody response as compared to polysaccharide vaccines. The human immunodeficiency virus (HIV) has been a curse in the humankind since decades. After years of research it is becoming more challenging to develop an effective vaccine against HIV. Question is whether this glycoconjugate vaccine can be a solution for this challenging disease. It was found that a good percentage of the broad neutralizing antibodies (bNAbs) in HIV-1 infected patients are against a dense high mannose region on envelope glycoprotein gp120 termed as high mannose patch (HMP) [26]. There have been many attempts to find out a suitable glycoconjugate vaccine with the principle of epitope-focusing targeting the HMP region of the HIV. McLellan et al. [27] identified that the PG9 antibodies made contacts with two glycans rich in mannose at Asn160 and Asn156 and a contiguous V1V2 (first and second variable loop of gp120) peptide b-strand. The other bNAbs including PGT121–123, 125–128 all target the V3 (third variable loop) region of gp120 [28, 29]. The V3 region of HIV-1 possesses three important N-linked glycosylation sites at the position N295, N332, N301 which are recognized by bNAbs. The synthetic V3 glycopeptide with high-mannose N-glycan at Asn332 was able to induce glycan dependent Ab responses in immunization studies in animals. In the follow-up experiment with a synthetic self adjuvating three-component immunogen made up of a 33-mer V3 glycopeptide epitope, a universal T-helper epitope P30, and a lipopeptide-based TLR-2 ligand showed glycan-dependent antibodies with a broader recognition of HIV-1 gp120 in comparison to the nonglycosylated V3 peptide. These observations indicating that the self adjuvating synthetic glycopeptide can be used as an important component to induce glycan-specific antibody response in HIV vaccine design [30]. Cancer is an another great havoc for the humankind. The tumor-associated carbohydrate antigens (TACAs) are considered as an important anticancer epitopes and have been targeted for anticancer glycoconjugate vaccines. Few of the TACA-based conjugate vaccines have reached randomized Phase III trials for melanoma, breast cancer, and nonsmall-cell lung cancer (including theratope, OPT822, GM2-KLH, racotumomab, and GD2-directed monoclonal Ab). On the other hand, the fully synthetic glycosphingolipid Globo-H epitope conjugated to CRM197 carrier was found to be more efficient in inducing IgG Ab production compared with KLH conjugates and also showed cross-reaction with Globo-H and Globo-H-related epitopes like SSEA3 and SSEA4 [31]. There is a high expression (around 100 times more than the normal) of mucin (MUC1) on the tumor cells, indicating MUC1 glycopeptides as an attractive target for cancer immunotherapy. Yin et al. [32] evaluated MUC1 peptides conjugated with bacteriophage Qb showed significant immune response against glycopeptides. In another study by Wu et al. [33], they have used a short synthetic Tn-nonapeptide of MUC1 (SAPDT*RPAP, * denotes glycosylation) conjugated with the bacteriophage Qb carrier showed higher anti-MUC1 IgG antibodies in immune-tolerant human MUC1 transgenic mice. These antibodies also showed high tumor binding and killing activities, good selectivity in glycopeptide recognition, and excellent recognition of human breast cancer over normal mammary tissues.

10. Conclusion

In the development of glycoconjugate vaccine, many factors play a crucial role such as saccharide size, carrier protein, conjugation chemistry and formulation. The methods are needed for faster identification of desired saccharide molecule on surface of pathogen, their characterization and their production in laboratory. The depth knowledge and extensive research of these factors will help in development of more effective glycoconjugate vaccines in short period of time. Moreover, we can expand their uses for cancer therapy. As we already have some licensed glycoconjugate vaccines for few infectious diseases, and for cancer therapy, there is ongoing phase lll trial; altogether we can see that this glycoconjugate vaccine has a great potential for some incurable disease conditions. In future to come up with effective glycoconjugate vaccines, we need more qualitative research and a good source of funding to solve the present disease scenario.

Conflict of interest

The authors declare no conflict of interest.

Abbreviations

Ab	antibody
APC	antigen presenting cell
AS	aluminum salt (Alum)
AUC	analytical ultracentrifugation
BCG	Bacillus Calmette Guérin
bNAbs	broad neutralizing antibodies
BSA	bovine serum albumin
CD	cluster of differentiation
CpG-ODN	cytosine phosphate guanosine oligodeoxynucleotides
CPS	capsular polysaccharide
CRM	cross reactive material
DNA	deoxyribonucleic acid
DT	diphtheria toxin
HA	hemagglutinin
Hib	*H. influenzae* type b
HIV	human immunodeficiency virus
HMP	high mannose patch
HPV	human papillomavirus
IgM	immunoglobulin M
LAM	lipoarabinomannan
LPS	lipopolysaccharide
MenB	meningococcus B
MHC	major histocompatibility complex
MPLA	monophosphorylated lipid A
mRNA	messenger ribonucleic acid
NMR	nuclear magnetic resonance
NOD	nucleotide oligomerization domain

OMPC	outer membrane protein complex
OMV	outer member vesicle
PCV	pneumococcal vaccine
PRP	polyribosyl ribitol phosphate
PRR	pattern recognition receptor
RIG-I	retinoic acid-inducible gene-I
ROS	reactive oxygen species
TACAs	tumor-associated carbohydrate antigens
TCV	typhoid conjugate vaccine
TT	tetanus toxoid
TLR	Toll-like receptor
VLP	virus like particle
WHO	World Health Organization

Author details

Fatema Akter[1]* and Sanjeev Kumar[2]

1 ICAR-Indian Veterinary Research Institute, Bareilly, Uttar Pradesh, India

2 Institute of Veterinary Sciences and Animal Husbandry, Siksha 'O' Anusandhan (Deemed to be University), Bhubaneswar, Odisha, India

*Address all correspondence to: dr.fatemaakter16@gmail.com

References

[1] Pollard AJ, Bijker EM. 2021. A guide to vaccinology: From basic principles to new developments. Nature Reviews Immunology. 2021;**21**(2):83-100

[2] Pulendran B, Ahmed R. Immunological mechanisms of vaccination. Nature Immunology. 2011;**12**(6):509-517

[3] Riddell NE. Immune Responses: Primary and Secondary. New Jersey, USA: eLS, John Wiley & Sons, Ltd; 2023. DOI: 10.1002/9780470015902.a0029196

[4] Alberts B, Johnson A, Lewis J, Raff M, Roberts K, Walter P. Lymphocytes and the cellular basis of adaptive immunity. In: Molecular Biology of the Cell. 4th ed. New York, USA: Garland Science; 2002

[5] Rappuoli R. Glycoconjugate vaccines: Principles and mechanisms. Science Translational Medicine. 2018;**10**:eaat4615

[6] Anderluh M, Berti F, Bzducha-Wrobel A, Chiodo F, Colombo C, Compostella F, et al. Recent advances on smart glycoconjugate vaccines in infections and cancer. The FEBS Journal. 2022;**289**:4251-4303

[7] MacCalman TE, Phillips-Jones MK, Harding SE. Glycoconjugate vaccines: Some observations on carrier and production methods. Biotechnology and Genetic Engineering Reviews. 2020;**35**:93-125. DOI: 10.1080/02648725.2019.1703614

[8] Liao G, Zhou Z, Liao J, Zu L, Wu Q, Guo Z. 6-O-branched oligo-β-glucanbased antifungal glycoconjugate vaccines. ACS Infectious Diseases. 2016;**2**:123-131

[9] Komarova BS, Orekhova MV, Tsvetkov YE, Beau R, Aimanianda V, Latgé JP, et al. Synthesis of a pentasaccharide & neoglycoconjugates related to fungal α-(1→3)-glucan & their use in the generation of antibodies to trace aspergillus fumigatus cell wall. Chemistry—A European Journal. 2015;**21**:1029-1035

[10] Adamo R, Hu QY, Torosantucci A, Crotti S, Brogioni G, Allan M, et al. Decipheringthestructure-immunogenicity relationship of anti-Candida glycoconjugate vaccines. Chemical Science. 2014;**5**:4302-4311

[11] Berti F, Ravenscroft N. Characterization of carbohydrate vaccines by NMR spectroscopy. In: Lepenies B, editor. Carbohydrate-Based Vaccines: Methods and Protocols Methods In Molecular Biology. Vol. 1331. New York, NY: Humana Press; 2015. pp. 189-209

[12] Harding SE, Abdelhameed AS, Gills RB, Morris GA, Adams GG. Characterization of capsular polysaccharies and their glycoconjugates by hydrodynamic methods. In: Lepenies B, editor. Carbohydrate-Based Vaccines: Methods and Protocols Methods In Molecular Biology. Vol. 1331. New York, NY: Humana Press; 2015. pp. 211-227

[13] Biemans R, Micoli F, Romano MR. Glycoconjugate vaccines, production and characterization. Recent Trends in Carbohydrate Chemistry. 2020;**2**:285-313. DOI: 10.1016/B978-0-12-820954-7.00008-6

[14] Togashi T, Mitsuya N, Kogawara O, Sumino S, Takanami Y, Sugizaki K. Immunogenicity & safety of a fully liquid aluminum phosphate adjuvanted

Haemophilus influenzae type b PRP-CRM197-conjugate vaccine in healthy Japanese children: A phase III, randomized, observer-blind, multicenter, parallel-group study. Vaccine. 2016;**34**:4635-4641

[15] Akeda Y, Koizumi Y, Takanami Y, Sumino S, Hattori Y, Sugizaki K, et al. Comparison of serum bactericidal & antibody titers induced by two Haemophilus influenzae type b conjugate vaccines: A phase III randomized double-blind study. Vaccine. 2018;**36**:1528-1532

[16] Chu RS, McCool T, Greenspan NS, Schreiber JR, Harding CV. CpG oligodeoxynucleotides act as adjuvants for pneumococcal polysaccharide-protein conjugate vaccines and enhance antipolysaccharide immunoglobulin G2a (IgG2a) and IgG3 antibodies. Infection and Immunity. 2000;**68**:1450-1456

[17] von Hunolstein C, Mariotti S, Teloni R, Alfarone G, Romagnoli G, Orefici G, et al. The adjuvant effect of synthetic oligodeoxynucleotide containing CpG motif converts the anti-haemophilus influenzae type b glycoconjugates into efficient antipolysaccharide and anti-carrier polyvalent vaccines. Vaccine. 2001;**19**:3058-3066

[18] Liao G, Zhou Z, Suryawanshi S, Mondal MA, Guo Z. Fully synthetic self-adjuvanting a-2,9- oligosialic acid based conjugate vaccines against group C meningitis. ACS Central Science. 2016;**2**:210-218

[19] Wang L, Feng S, Wang S, Li H, Guo Z, Gu G. Synthesis and immunological comparison of differently linked lipoarabinomannan oligosaccharidemonophosphoryl lipid A conjugates as antituberculosis vaccines. Journal of Organic Chemistry. 2017;**82**:12085-12096

[20] Deng S, Bai L, Reboulet R, Matthew R, Engler DA, Teyton L, et al. A peptidefree, liposome-based oligosaccharide vaccine, adjuvanted with a natural killer T cell antigen, generates robust antibody responses in vivo. Chemical Science. 2014;**5**:1437-1441

[21] Hassane FS, Phalipon A, Tanguy M, Guerreiro C, Belot F, Frisch B, et al. Rational design and immunogenicity of liposomebased diepitope constructs: Application to synthetic oligosaccharides mimicking the Shigella flexneri 2a Oantigen. Vaccine. 2009;**27**:5419-5426

[22] Borja-Tabora CFC, Montalban C, Memish ZA, Boutriau D, Kolhe D, Miller JM, et al. Long-term immunogenicity & safety after a single dose of the quadrivalent meningococcal serogroups A, C, W, & Y tetanus toxoid conjugate vaccine in adolescents & adults: 5-year follow-up of an open, randomized trial. BMC Infectious Diseases. 2015;**15**:409

[23] Holme D, Findlow H, Sow SO, Idoko OT, Preziosi MP, Carlone G, et al. Neisseria meningitidis Group A IgG1 & IgG2 subclass immune response in African children aged 12-23 months following meningococcal vaccination. Clinical Infectios Diseases. 2015;**61**:563-569

[24] Ramasamy MN, Clutterbuck EA, Haworth K, Bowman J, Omar O, Thompson AJ, et al. Randomized clinical trial to evaluate the immunogenicity of quadrivalent meningococcal conjugate & polysaccharide vaccines in adults in the United Kingdom. Clinical Vaccine Immunology. 2014;**21**:1164-1168

[25] Rothstein EP, Schiller RP, Girone JA, Hipp TJ, Souder RL, Bernstein HH,

et al. Response of 7- to 15-month-old infants to sequential immunization with Haemophilus influenzae type b-CRM197 conjugate & polysaccharide vaccines. American Journal of Diseases of Children. 1991;**1991**(145):898-900

[26] Berndsen ZT, Chakraborty S, Wang X, Cottrell CA, Torres JL, Diedrich JK, et al. Visualization of the HIV-1 Env glycan shield across scales. The Proceedings of the National Academy of Sciences. 2020;**117**:28014-28025

[27] McLellan JS, Pancera M, Carrico C, Gorman J, Julien J-P, Khayat R, et al. Structure of HIV-1 Gp120 V1/V2 domain with broadly neutralizing antibody PG9. Nature. 2011;**480**:336-343

[28] Pejchal R, Doores KJ, Walker LM, Khayat R, Huang P-S, Wang S-K, et al. A potent and broad neutralizing antibody recognizes and penetrates the HIV glycan shield. Science. 2011;**334**:1097-1103

[29] Walker LM, Huber M, Doores KJ, Falkowska E, Pejchal R, Julien J-P, et al. Broad neutralization coverage of HIV by multiple highly potent antibodies. Nature. 2011;**477**:466-470

[30] Cai H, Orwenyo J, Giddens JP, Yang Q, Zhang R, LaBranche CC, et al. Synthetic three-component HIV-1 V3 glycopeptide immunogens induce glycan-dependent antibody responses. Cell Chemical Biology. 2017;**24**:1513-1522

[31] Huang Y-L, Hung J-T, Cheung SKC, Lee H-Y, Chu K-C, Li S-T, et al. Carbohydrate-based vaccines with a glycolipid adjuvant for breast cancer. The Proceedings of the National Academy of Sciences. 2013;**110**:2517-2522

[32] Yin Z, Wu X, Kaczanowska K, Sungsuwan S, Aragones MC, Pett C, et al. Antitumor humoral and T cell responses by mucin-1 conjugates of bacteriophage Qb in wild-type mice. ACS Chemical Biology. 2018;**13**:1668-1676

[33] Wu X, Yin Z, McKay C, Pett C, Yu J, Schorlemer M, et al. Protective epitope discovery and design of MUC1-based vaccine for effective tumor protections in immunotolerant mice. Journal of the American Chemical Society. 2018;**140**:16596-16609

Section 2

Management of Global Diseases

Chapter 5

MFG-E8, A Novel Biomarker for Alzheimer's Disease and Its Amyloidotic Feature

Hitoshi Sohma, Michitoshi Kimura, Ayaka Sudo, Mihoko Ohashi, Hiromi Hamano and Yasuo Kokai

Abstract

Biomarker study on dementia has developed and the most reliable fluid markers are amyloid peptide (Aβ), TAU, and phosphorylated TAU detected in cerebrospinal fluid (CSF). We have focused on novel Alzheimer's disease (AD) biomarker candidates (annexin A5 and Milk fat globule-EGF factor 8 protein [MFG-E8]), Ca^{2+} and phospholipid binding properties, which were elevated in the neuronal cell culture medium by $A\beta_{42}$ treatment. We have previously reported annexin A5 as an AD biomarker. In this chapter, we focused on MFG-E8. An immunohistochemical study using AD mouse model (APP/PS1) brains revealed characteristic distributions of the staining with anti-MFG-E8 antibody. Anti-MFG-E8 antibody staining was detected in the core regions of the anti-Aβ-antibody stained plaques in 20 weeks old and older APP/PS1 mice, while no staining was observed in control (wild mouse) and anti-Aβ-antibody staining was detected outside of it. The volume of the staining was augmented with advancing age. It was further revealed that the MFG-E8 protein changed to amyloidotic features over time from the Congo red spectral peak shift and electron microscopic study in vitro. As the emergence of senile plaque takes a long time, MFG-E8 present in the plaque might be in an amyloidotic form. From these results, MFG-E8 is a novel biomarker candidate for AD.

Keywords: Alzheimer's disease, biomarker, MFG-E8, amyloid, immunohistochemistry, Congo red, electron microscopy

1. Introduction

Accumulating data of biomarker study for Alzheimer's disease (AD) show that the cerebrospinal fluid (CSF) biomarkers [amyloid β peptides, total tau (T-tau), and phosphorylated tau (P-tau)] are significant elements of AD pathophysiology, which has been confirmed from the clinical research. On the other hand, although many blood biomarkers have been suggested, reliable biomarker is scarce at present compared with CSF biomarkers.

We have been engaged in Alzheimer biomarker studies, especially blood plasma biomarkers. To identify biomarker candidates for AD, we prepared primary culture neuronal cells from mice embryos and isolated the proteins increased in culture media by $A\beta_{42}$-treatment, possibly secreted proteins, using a proteomic approach [1]. Since plasma biomarkers are expected to be blood–brain barrier permeable, we focused on lipid-binding proteins. For the isolation of biomarker candidates, we prepared phosphatidylserine (PS) binding proteins using a unique method with our original synthetic thermoresponsive magnetic nanoparticles (Therma-max, Magnabeat, Chiba, Japan) coated with PS, denoted as nanoliposome [2]. As PS is exposed to the outer membrane of cells during the apoptotic process, PS-binding proteins may be involved in neuronal damage and might become plasma biomarkers. Lipid-coated nanoliposomes, a mimic of liposomes, disperse well at low temperatures such as at 4°C and aggregate at room temperature, and stick to a magnet, which is a simple method [3]. Using this method, we isolated the Ca^{2+} fraction which was released with EGTA. As $A\beta_{42}$-dependent cytotoxicity involves disruption of Ca^{2+} homeostasis, we focused on the proteins involved in Ca^{2+} signaling, Ca^{2+} binding proteins. Among the proteins identified, we have previously focused on annexin A5 as a biomarker candidate [1]. We have shown that secretion of annexin A5 was augmented in the neuronal culture model and that it was significantly increased in plasma from both mouse model and AD patients, compared with control and published several papers [1, 4, 5]. In addition to annexin A5, we also have been interested in another candidate, Milk fat globule EGF factor 8 (MFG-E8) having PS and Ca^{2+}-binding properties [2]. MFG-E8, known as lactadherin, is a secreted glycoprotein originally identified as a component of milk fat globules [6]. MFG-E8 is expressed and secreted by a variety of cells and tissues such as macrophages and dendritic cells. It was shown that MFG-E8 plays a role in the activation of engulfment by phagocytic cells with its specific binding sites for both apoptotic cell membrane and phagocytic cell [6, 7]. It was reported that MFG-E8 interacted with $A\beta$ peptides, and also had a role in the activation of $A\beta_{42}$ phagocytosis by brain cells in vitro [8–10]. In our previous study using the AD mouse model (TG2576), we identified the distinctive localization of MFG-E8, in the center of amyloid plaque [2]. In this chapter, using another mouse model (APP/PS1) we report the time-dependent pattern of immuno-staining of MFG-E8 and the unique physical property of MFG-E8 (amyloidotic) in vitro, with Congo red (CR) spectrophotometry and electron microgram. Formation of amyloidogenic proteins characteristic to neurodegenerative disorders, such as AD, and dementia with Lewy body [11, 12]. Thus, MFG-E8 might be a novel marker having amyloidotic properties.

2. Materials and methods

2.1 Reagents

Ultrapure grade CR was purchased from Merck KGaA (Darmstadt, German). Human recombinant MFG-E8 (rMFG-E8) was purchased from R&D Systems, Inc. (Minneapolis, MN, USA). 3, 3′-diaminobenzizine (DAB) was purchased from Tokyo Chemical Industry Co. Ltd. (Tokyo, Japan). Collodion film on the TEM grids (200 mesh) was purchased from Nisshin EM Co., Ltd. (Tokyo, Japan).

2.2 Antibody

Armenian hamster monoclonal antibody against mouse MFG-E8 and goat polyclonal antibody against Armenian hamster IgG were purchased from Medical

& Biological Laboratories Co. (Nagoya, Japan). Mouse monoclonal antibody (IgG) against human amyloid β, mouse monoclonal antibody against human MFG-E8, and HRP-conjugated rabbit anti-mouse IgG (H+L) were purchased from Immuno-Biological Laboratories Co. Ltd. (Gunma, Japan). Alexa Fluoro™594-conjugated donkey anti-mouse IgG and DyLight™488-conjugated goat anti-Armenian hamster IgG were from BioLegend (Tokyo, Japan).

2.3 Animals

Alzheimer model mice (APP/PS1), double transgenic mice expressing a chimeric mouse/human amyloid precursor protein (Mo/HuAPP695swe), and a mutant human presenilin 1 (PS1-dE9) were purchased from The Jackson Laboratories (Bar Harbor, ME, USA). This project was approved by the Sapporo Medical University Animal Experimental Ethics Committee (the authorization numbers: 11-011 and 14-014).

2.4 Immunohistochemistry

For immunohistochemistry (IHC) staining, formalin-fixed paraffin-embedded mouse brain sections (either 4 or 10 μm thick) were deparaffinized with xylene and treated with 0.3% H_2O_2, and then incubated in Histofine (Nichirei Biosciences Inc., Tokyo Japan) with microwave (500 W) for 10 minutes for antigen activation. The sections were then incubated in 70% formic acid for 5 minutes and Bloc Ace (KAC Co., Ltd., Tokyo, Japan) for 1 hour when HRP-labeled secondary antibody was used for visualization. The sections were incubated with 5% FBS in 4% Bloc Ace for blocking, and then with primary antibodies diluted with 4% Bloc Ace in PBS (1:100 for both anti-Aβ and anti-MFG-E8 antibodies) overnight at 4°C. The primary antibody binding was then detected by incubating the sections with HRP-labeled secondary antibody [anti-mouse IgG (1:400 dilution) or anti-Armenian hamster antibody (1:6000 dilution)], or, DyLight 488-conjugated anti-mouse antibody (1:30 dilution) and Alexa 594-conjugated anti-Armenian hamster antibody (1:30 dilution) for 45 minutes at room temperature. Antibody visualization was done with DAB for HRP-labeled secondary antibodies. For observing fluorescently labeled sections after final washing in PBS, they were mounted with VECTASIELD containing 4′, 6-diamidino-2 phenylindole (DAPI) (VECTOR, Burlingame, CA, USA) and used confocal microscopy (LSM520 META, Zeiss, Tokyo, Japan). Fluorescent images were acquired with laser lines 405, 488, and 543 nm using bandpass filters 420–480, 505–530, and 560–605 nm, respectively.

2.5 Congo red spectral shift assay for amyloid (spectrophotometry)

CR is a well-known for histological stain to verify the presence of amyloidal deposits in tissue. The binding of CR to amyloid has since been characterized and shown to depend on the secondary conformation of the amyloid, the β-pleated sheet conformation. In the present study, about 200 μM CR stock solution was prepared by dissolving in a solution of 90% phosphate-buffered saline (PBS) and 10% ethanol and filtered twice through a cellulose acetate membrane (pore size 0.45 μm) and stored at room temperature. Determination of the accurate concentration of CR stock solution was done by measuring the absorbance of a diluted aliquot in a solution of 1 mM sodium phosphate (pH 7.0) and 40% ethanol with ε_{505} of 5.94×10^4/cm·M. Absorption spectra were collected by a Shimadzu UV-2550 double-beam spectrophotometer with a

UV-enhanced quartz cell. For analyzing peak shift by CR binding to protein, 64 μg/ml rMFG-E8 in PBS and 0.02% NaN_3 was mixed with 3 μM CR, preincubated at room temperature for 15 minutes, and the spectrum was collected. CR and protein mixture solution was placed in the sample cell and PBS in the reference cell. We also collected different spectra in that the CR and protein mixture was placed in the sample cell and CR alone was in the reference cell.

2.6 Electron microscopy

Aliquots of rMFG-E8 solution dissolved in PBS and 0.01% NaN_3 were placed on a Collodion film on the TEM grids, and let sit for 10 minutes at room temperature. The solution that remained on the film was adsorbed with filter paper and the film was air-dried. Staining was done with a 4% uranyl acetate for 1 minute. After washing with H_2O and air-died, samples were viewed under a transmission electron microscope (JEM-1400, JEO Tokyo, Japan).

3. Results

3.1 Immunohistochemical studies on mouse brain

In this study, to explore the localization of MFG-E8 in the brain we used double transgenic mice (APP/PS1) expressing a chimeric mutant mouse/human amyloid precursor protein and a mutant human presenilin 1, both directed to CNS neurons. As these mutations are associated with early-onset AD, APP/PS1 mice have been widely used in studying neurological disorders of the brain, specifically AD and amyloid plaque formation. From the IHC study anti-Aβ-antibody stained spots, (amyloid plaques) were observed at 20 weeks old and older mice (**Figure 1**). Characteristically, the anti-Aβ antibody stained plaques with larger radiuses developed in older mice (**Figure 1**). On the other hand, no staining was observed in control (wild type) mice even at 40 months old (data not shown). It is noticeable that the staining with anti-MFG-E8 antibody was also observed at 20 weeks old and older mice (**Figure 2**) whereas no staining was observed in control (wild type) mice (data not shown), which seems similar to the pattern of the anti-Aβ antibody stained plaques although the intensity of staining was weak.

To further explore the localization of both Aβ and MFG-E8, we next performed immunofluorescent staining (double staining) and observed specimens with confocal laser microscopy. The immuno-stained pattern with both anti-Aβ and anti-MFG-E8 antibodies shows a characteristic pattern. Anti-MFG-E8 antibody was detected in the core region and anti-Aβ antibody was detected in the outer side of MFG-E8 in all plaques identified (**Figure 3**), and partly overlapping (yellow) sites were observed. Relatively, the magnitude of the anti-MFG-E8 antibody staining core region was larger in older mice compared with younger ones. On the other hand, no anti-MFG-E8 antibody staining was observed in wild-type mice (control) (data not shown). The characteristic localization of both Aβ and MFG-E8 was well shown in the 3D reconstruction image (**Figure 3**).

3.2 Congo red spectrum shift by MFG-E8

Particular amyloidogenic proteins have been reported in neurodegenerative diseases such as Aβ for AD and α-synuclein for Dementia with Lewy bodies [11]. It is well

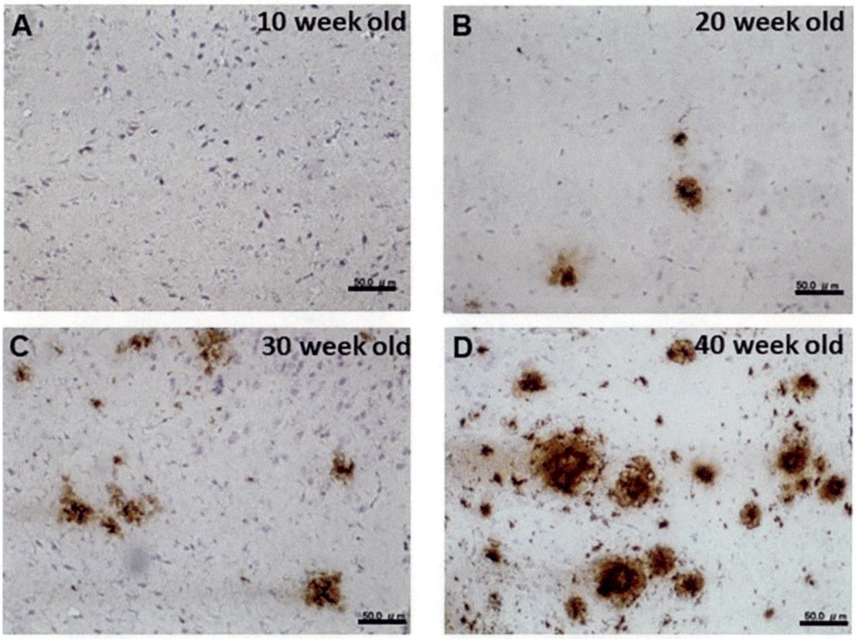

Figure 1.
Immunohistochemical staining of APP/PS1 mouse brain (Aβ). Antibody visualization was done with DAB. A. 10 weeks old; B. 20 weeks old; C. 30 weeks old; D. 40 weeks old. Bars in the insets show 50 μm.

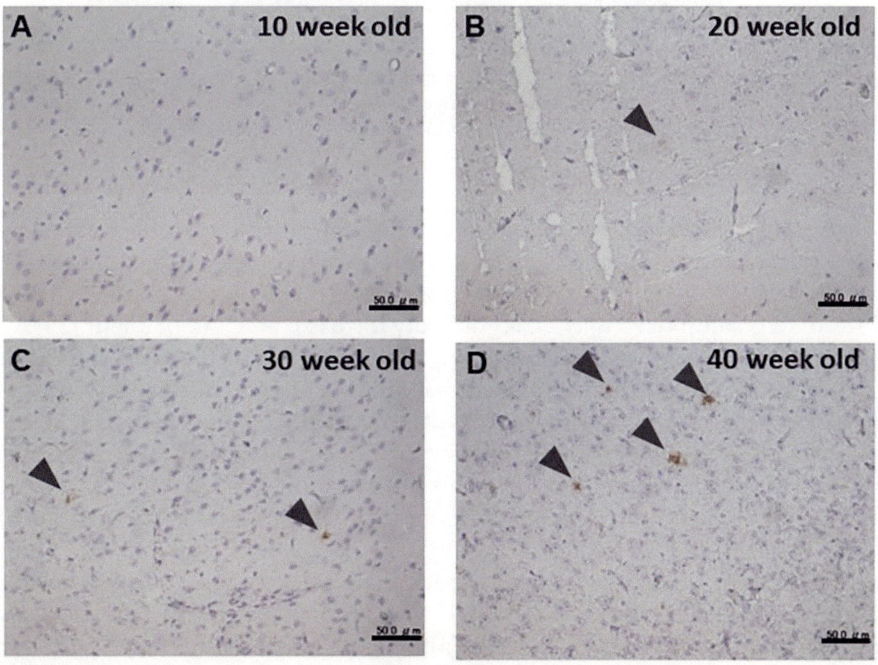

Figure 2.
Immunohistochemical staining of APP/PS1 mouse brain (MFG-E8). Antibody visualization was done with DAB. A. 10 weeks old; B. 20 weeks old; C. 30 weeks old; D. 40 weeks old. Bars in the insets show 50 μm.

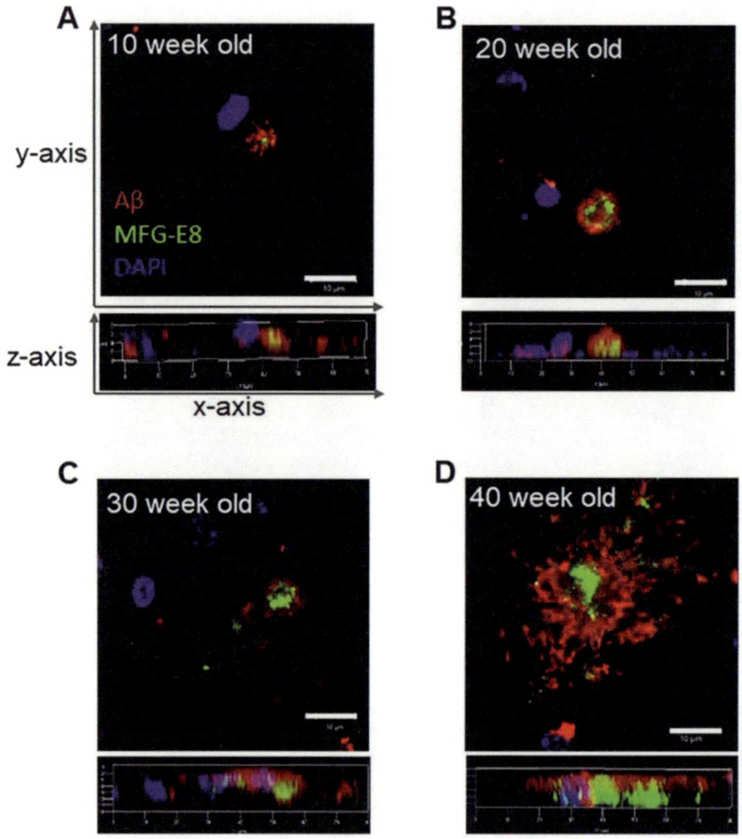

Figure 3.
Fluorescent immunohistochemical staining of APP/PS1 mouse brain (MFG-E8). Fluorescently labeled antibodies against Aβ and MFG-E8 are shown in red and green, respectively. For nuclear staining, DAPI is included in an aqueous anti-fade mounting medium, which shows in blue. A. 10 weeks old; B. 20 weeks old; C. 30 weeks old; D. 40 weeks old. Bars in the insets show 10 μm.

known that Aβ peptide is a major component in senile plaque and it forms amyloid, whose physicochemical and biological properties have been elucidated and published in many papers [13, 14]. In vitro study demonstrated that when Aβ peptide with 40 or 42 residues is solubilized in H_2O, it gradually forms an amyloid filament [15]. CR, a well-known histological stain, is extensively used to reveal the presence of amyloidal deposits in tissue. It is also demonstrated that binding of CR to the amyloid form of Aβ peptide caused specific spectral peak shifts of CR in vitro (redshift) [13, 14]. It is plausible that the secondary conformation of the amyloid specifically contributes to the spectral change. CR peak shift was also used for the quantitative assay of the amyloid form of Aβ peptide [13]. Based on these findings, we next analyzed the CR spectrum with rMFG-E8. As amyloid formation takes place taking time, we compared the spectra of rMFG-E8 with different pre-incubation times: short-term (2 hours) and long-term (14 days) incubation at 37°C after lyophilized rMFG-E8 was dissolved. Interestingly, the maximum peak around 500 nm of the spectrum of rMFG-E8 after 14-day incubation shifted to a longer wavelength (redshift) compared with that after 2 hours pre-incubated MFG-E8 (**Figure 4**). The difference spectra show the peak shift more clearly. These results suggest that MFG-E8 is an amyloidotic protein.

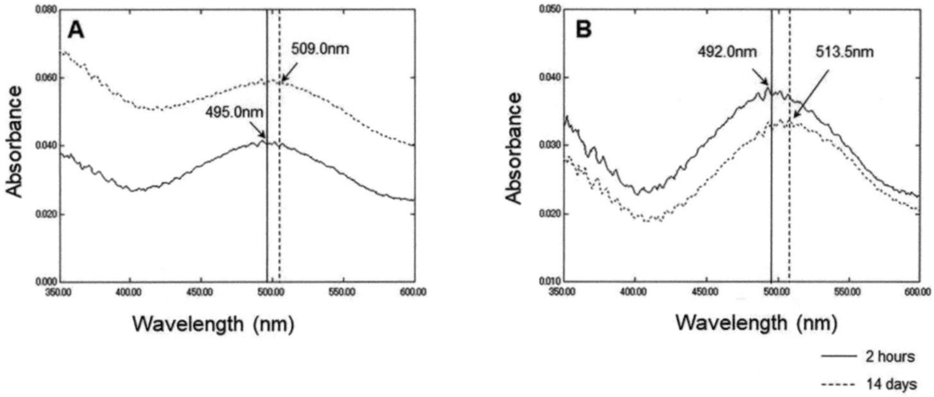

Figure 4.
CR spectrum shift assay of MFG-E8. A. Absorbance spectrum of CR with MFG-E8 after pre-incubation for 2 hours or 14 days. B. Different absorbance spectrum between CR with MFG-E8 after pre-incubation for 2 hours or 14 days, and CR alone. Vertical lines in the insets show the maximum wavelengths of each spectrum.

3.3 Electron microscopic analysis of MFG-E8

Negative staining transmission electron micrograms of rMFG-E8 solution pre-incubated for 2 hours, 14 days, and 21 days after dissolving were compared. It was shown that fibrous aggregates appeared in the rMFG-E8 solutions pre-incubated for 14 and 21 days, whereas much less fibrous aggregates in the rMFG-E8 solution after 2 hours incubation (**Figure 5**). Thus, electron microscopy also reveals that rMFG-E8 is likely to form amyloidotic form over time.

Taking the results of CR spectral peak shift in 14-day preincubated rMFG-E8 into account, it is conceivable that the rMFG-E8 whole molecule is an amyloidotic protein.

4. Discussion

In our previous study, we explored brain MFG-E8 using an AD model mice (tg2576) [2]. IHC study with tg2576 mice at 12 months old revealed that the staining

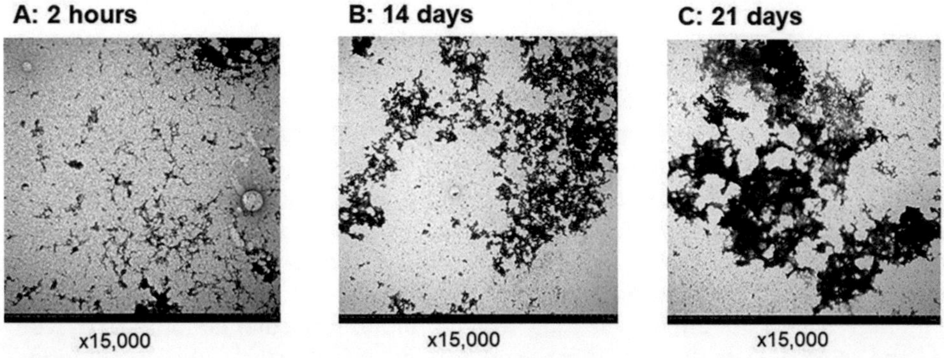

Figure 5.
Electron microscopic analysis of rMFG-E8 (negative staining). Electron microgram of rMFG-E8 after different times pre-incubation. Pre-incubation times are as follows: A. 2 hours; B. 14 weeks; C. 21 weeks.

pattern with anti-MFG-E8 antibody was similar to that with APP/PS1 mice ([2] and **Figure 1**). Immuno-staining with the antibody was observed in the core region of the senile plaques in both tg2576 and APP/PS1. In the present study, we further demonstrated with APP/PS1 mice that localization of the anti-MFG-E8 antibody staining was observed in the core region of the plaques that emerged from the early stage (20 weeks old) (**Figures 1** and **2**). All areas stained with anti-MFG-E8 antibodies have always anti-Aβ antibodies staining areas (**Figure 3**). The characteristic localization of MFG-E8 might suggest that MFG-E8 plays a role in the formation of plaque. In this study, as the plaque was identified by anti-Aβ-antibody staining, it is uncertain whether or not the emergence of MFG-E8 in the plaque was a preceding event to the assembling of Aβ.

The radius of plaque in older mice relatively becomes more extensive over time. The anti-MFG-E8 antibody-stained regions, the cores of the plaques, also become more extensive, suggesting that accumulation of MFG-E8 took place in the core regions during the growth of plaque. As amyloid forms with homogeneous proteins, there might exist an unknown mechanism for growing MFG-E8 only in the core region when MFG-E8 is secreted. In the present study, MFG-E8 was shown to have an amyloidotic property (**Figures 4** and **5**). As rMFG-E8 used in this study was prepared from secreted mammalian cells, freshly dissolved rMFG-E8 is not likely to be amyloidotic. It was also shown amyloidotic aggregates of MFG-E8 were observed after 14 days in this study. The formation of amyloid plaques requires a long time in the brain. Thus, MFG-E8 in plaque is in amyloidotic conformation. The amyloidotic feature of MFG-E8 might be favorable in part for the specific location in the plaque. Many constituents in the plaque have been identified [16, 17], but MFG-E8 has not been reported before.

Medin is an integral fragment derived from MFG-E8, which was first found in aortic smooth muscle cells over 50 years of age [18, 19]. Medin, a 5.5 kDa component located in the MFG-E8 FF5/8-C2 domain, contains the amino acid sequence favorable for amyloid formation [18, 20]. Recently medin amyloid in blood vessels was shown to cause cerebrovascular dysfunction in aged mice [21]. It was further shown the medin co-localized with vascular Aβ in the AD mouse model and the vascular Aβ deposition was reduced in the medin-deficient mice [22]. In the present study, MFG-E8 was shown to localize in the senile plaque (**Figure 3**). Moreover, rMFG-E8 was suggested to make an amyloidotic form in time (**Figures 4** and **5**). Even after 14 days of incubation, no fragment was observed on SDS PAGE (data not shown). Thus, both CR peak shift and electron microscopic image suggest an amyloidotic conformation of a whole molecule of rMFG-E8. Although it is not certain if the immunostained MFG-E8 in the plaque contained a fragment of MFG-E8 or not, either form of MFG-E8 possibly exists in the plaque.

On the other hand, MFG-E8 was initially identified as a component of milk fat globules and indicated to have a role in pathological and physiological processes, including the clearance of apoptotic cells and angiogenesis [23]. It was also suggested that MFG-E8 has a protective role against Aβ-dependent toxicity in the cell cultural assay [8, 9]. These results indicate that secreted MFG-E8, not amyloidotic form, is likely to have a protective role. It has been demonstrated that medin enhances various reactive oxygen species and reactive nitrogen species produced by both endothelial cells and vascular smooth muscle cells, which promotes vascular endothelial dysfunction and arterial stiffening [24]. On the other hand, it is obscure if the amyloidotic MFG-E8 has a role pathologically or physiologically.

It has been reported that MFG-E8 in the brain was identified in the vasculature but not in plaque-rich areas [10]. In contrast, the present study suggested the localization of MFG-E8 in the core region in plaques by anti-MFG-E8 antibody staining. The reason for the discrepancy between our results and other reports is uncertain.

A significant decrease in MFG-E8 mRNA was reported in AD patients [8]. On the other hand, our previous in vitro study showed an increase in MFG-8 by $A\beta_{42}$ treatment. In the present study, the magnitude of the area of anti-MFG-E8 antibody staining was increased in older mice, while no staining by the anti-MFG-E8 antibody was detected in the control. These findings may indicate that the production and secretion of MFG-E8 increased or that the clearance of MFG-E8 was attenuated in older APP/PS1 mice. It has been elucidated that the disruption of Ca^{2+} homeostasis can lead to widespread impairment of cellular and synaptic signaling, subsequently contributing to dementia including AD [25]. It might be possible that MFG-E8 detected in plaques (outer of cells) was relevant to cell damage.

Previously, we demonstrated that annexin A5 is a potential plasma biomarker. Annexin A5 was reported to be able to cross the blood–brain barrier [26], in which annexin's lipid binding properties may be favorable for crossing. It is conceivable that MFG-E8 may also cross the blood–brain barrier due to its phospholipid-binding properties. Our previous results suggest that the blood level of MFG-E8 in AD patients was higher than in control, although the number of samples was limited [2]. In spite of that MFG-E8 is an amyloidotic protein and it requires time for amyloidotic fiber (a high molecular mass aggregate) formation, it is plausible that a fraction of MFG-E8 might cross the blood–brain barrier after secretion from brain cells. In the next step, we would like to investigate further the verification of MFG-E8 as a blood biomarker.

Author details

Hitoshi Sohma[1,2*], Michitoshi Kimura[3], Ayaka Sudo[1], Mihoko Ohashi[2], Hiromi Hamano[1] and Yasuo Kokai[2]

1 Department of Educational Development, Sapporo Medical University Center for Medical Education, Sapporo, Japan

2 Department of Biomedical Engineering, Sapporo Medical University School of Medicine, Sapporo, Japan

3 Division of Morphological Research, Sapporo Medical University Biomedical Research Center, Sapporo, Japan

*Address all correspondence to: sohma@sapmed.ac.jp

References

[1] Yamaguchi M, Kokai Y, Imai S, Utsumi K, Matsumoto K, Honda H, et al. Investigation of annexin A5 as a biomarker for Alzheimer's disease using neuronal cell culture and mouse model. Journal of Neuroscience Research. 2010;**88**:2682-2692

[2] Kimura M, Sohma H, Matsuki K, Yamaguchi M, Imai S, Kokai Y. Milk fat globule-EGF-factor 8 is induced from neuronal cells upon stimulation of Aβ oligomer and specifically localizes in amyloid plaques in the brain of mouse model for Alzheimer's disease. Sapporo Medical Journal. 2017;**85**(supplement):23-34

[3] Ohnishi N, Furukawa H, Hata H, Wang J-M, An C-I, Fukusaki E, et al. High-efficiency bioaffinity of cells and proteins using novel thermoresponsive biotinylated magnetic nanoparticles. NanoBiotechnology. 2006;**2**:43-49

[4] Sohma H, Imai S, Takei N, Honda H, Matsumoto K, Utsumi K, et al. Evaluation of annexin A5 as a biomarker for Alzheimer's disease and dementia with Lewy bodies. Frontiers in Aging Neuroscience. 2013;**5**:1-7

[5] Sohma H, Kokai Y. Plasma Biomarkers in Alzheimer's Disease. London, UK: InTechOpen; 2016

[6] Aziz M, Jacob A, Matsuda A, Wang P. Review: Milk fat globule-EGF factor 8 expression, function and plausible signal transduction in resolving inflammation. Apoptosis. 2011;**16**:1077-1086

[7] Yi Y-S. Functional role of milk fat globule-epidermal growth factor VIII in macrophage-mediated inflammatory responses and inflammatory/autoimmune diseases. Mediators of Inflammation (Hindawi Publishing Corporation). 2016;**2016**:12. Article ID 5628486. DOI: 10.1155/2016/5628486

[8] Boddaert J, Kinugawa K, Lambert J-C, Boukhtouche F, Zoll J, Merval R, et al. Evidence of a role for lactadherin in Alzheimer's disease. The American Journal of Pathology. 2007;**170**:921-929

[9] Li E, Noda M, Doi Y, Parajuli B, Kawanokuchi J, Sonobe Y, et al. The neuroprotective effects of milk fat globule-EGF factor 8 against oligomeric amyloid β toxicity. Journal of Neuroinflammation. 2012;**9**:148. Available from: http://www.jneuroinflammation.com/content/9/1/148

[10] Marazuela P, Solé M, Bonaterra-Pastra A, Pizarro J, Camacho J, Martínez-Sáez E, et al. MFG-E8 (LACTADHERIN): A novel marker associated with cerebral amyloid angiopathy. Acta Neuropathologica Communications. 2021;**9**(145):1-17

[11] Irwin DJ, Hurtig HI. The contribution of Tau, amyloid-beta and alpha-synuclein pathology to dementia in Lewy body disorders. Journal of Alzheimers Disease and Parkinsonism. 2018;**8**:1-13

[12] Zerovnik E, Stoka V, Mirtic A, Guncar G, Grdadolnik J, Staniforth RA, et al. Mechanisms of amyloid fibril formation – focus on domain-swapping. The FEBS Journal. 2011;**278**:2263-2282

[13] Klunk WE, Jacob RF, Mason RP. Quantitating amyloid by Congo red spectral shift assay. Methods in Enzymology. 1999;**309**:285-305

[14] Yokoyama K, Fisher AD, Amori AR, Welchons DR, McKnight RE.

Spectroscopic and calorimetric studies of Congo red dye-amyloid β peptide complexes. Journal of Biophysical Chemistry. 2010;**1**(3):153-163

[15] Finder VH, Glockshuber R. Amyloid-β aggregation. Neurodegenerative Diseases. 2007;**4**:13-27

[16] Liao L, Cheng D, Wang J, Duong DM, Losik TG, Gearing M, et al. Proteomic characterization of postmortem Amyloid plaques isolated by laser capture microdissection. The Journal of Biological Chemistry. 2004;**279**:37061-37068

[17] Rahman MM, Lendel C. Extracellular protein components of amyloid plaques and their roles in Alzheimer's disease pathology. Neurodegeneration. 2021;**16**:59. DOI: 10.1186/s13024-021-00465-0

[18] Haeggqvist B, Naeslund J, Sletten K, Westermark GT, Mucchiano G, Tjernberg LO, et al. Medin: An integral fragment of aortic smooth muscle cell-produced lactadherin forms the most common human amyloid. Proceedings of the National Academy of Sciences of the United States of America. 1999;**96**:8669-8674

[19] Peng S, Westermark GT, Naeslund J, Haeggqvist B, Glennert J, Westermark P. Medin and medin-amyloid in aging inflamed and non-inflamed temporal arteries. Journal of Pathology. 2002;**196**:91-96

[20] Larsson A, Söderberg L, Westermark GT, Sletten K, Engström U, Tjernberg LO, et al. Unwinding fibril formation of medin, the peptide of the most common form of human amyloid. Biochemical and Biophysical Research Communications. 2007;**361**:822-828

[21] Degenhardt K, Wagner J, Skodras A, Candlish M, Koppelmann AJ, Wild K, et al. Medin aggregation causes cerebrovascular dysfunction in aging wild-type mice. Proceedings of the National Academy of Sciences. 2020;**117**:23925-23931

[22] Wagner J, Degenhardt K, Veit M, Louros N, Konstantoulea K, Skodras A, et al. Medin co-aggregates with vascular amyloid-β in Alzheimer's disease. Nature. 2022;**612**:123-131

[23] Hanayama R, Tanaka M, Miwa K, Shinohara A, Iwamatsu A, Nagata S. Identification of a factor that links apoptotic cells to phagocytes. Nature. 2002;**417**:182-187

[24] Wang M, McGrawand KR, Monticone RE. Milk fat globule epidermal growth factor VIII fragment medin in age-associated arterial adverse remodeling and arterial disease. Cells. 2023;**12**:253. DOI: 10.3390/cells12020253

[25] Cascella R, Cecch C. Calcium dyshomeostasis in Alzheimer's disease pathogenesis. International Journal of Molecular Sciences. 2021;**22**:4914. DOI: 10.3390/ijms22094914

[26] Caserta MT, Caccioppo D, Lapin GD, Ragin A, Groothuis DR. Blood-brain barrier integrity in Alzheimer's disease patients and elderly control subjects. Journal of Neuropsychiatry and Clinical Neurosciences. 1998;**10**:78-84

Chapter 6

The Link between Hypouricemia and Neurodegenerative Disorders

Anna Mihailova, Maximiliane Trapp and Natalija Kakurina

Abstract

The potential danger to patients' health due to hypouricemia has only recently become a research topic of interest. While it has been established that normal uric acid levels have antioxidative and neuroprotective properties, the loss of these functions with uric acid levels below the normal range have been studied only recently and findings suggest potential detrimental effects on the brain and cognitive abilities. The purpose of this study is to look at potential connections between hypouricemia and neurodegenerative disorders such as Alzheimer's disease and vascular dementia. Seventy-seven inpatients and outpatients with routine uric acid testing were included and further stratified into patients with neurodegenerative disease and patients without neurodegenerative disease. The results showed that rates of Alzheimer's disease differ between patients with hypouricemia and normal uric acid levels, however this association was not found for patients with vascular dementia. This provides evidence for potential effects of hypouricemia and raises the question for further research define a safe range of serum uric acid.

Keywords: uric acid, hypouricemia, neurodegenerative diseases, Alzheimer's disease, vascular dementia

1. Introduction

The effects of hyperuricemia on the cardiovascular system have been extensively studied and it is widely known that hyperuricemia is regarded as a risk factor for cardiovascular disease such as hypertension. Hypouricemia, on the other hand, had been mostly disregarded in research until recently when researchers started to investigate potential sequela from below normal uric acid levels. This was mostly due to the advent of newer and more effective urate lowering medication that it raised the question whether lowering uric acid below normal levels could have any clinical significance.

1.1 The uric acid paradox

Uric acid had been studied in the vitro where it was established that normal levels have oxidative properties that are pro-inflammatory within cells and antioxidative and neuroprotective effects by reducing oxidative stress within plasma to which the discovering researchers referred to as the oxidative-antioxidative paradox. This aligns with the findings that hyperuricemia can have an inflammatory response causing pathologies such as gout and cardiovascular disease through endothelial dysfunction while hypouricemia could have potential effects on the neurovascular system by the loss of the antioxidative and neuroprotective properties. And indeed, recent suggest exactly this finding that there could be a possible association between low serum uric acid levels and the development of neurodegenerative diseases. Researchers are now interested in finding evidence that preventing uric acid levels to fall below the normal range could ultimately prevent neurodegenerative diseases and if so, what would a safe range of uric acid levels be.

This work embraces a review of articles and recent research on hypouricemia that had been published between November 1980 until November 2019 and investigates a patient group with neurodegenerative disease and a patient group without such a disease for possible differences. The aim was to explore a possible relationship between subnormal uric acid levels and neurodegenerative disease among patients in Latvia.

2. Uric acid and its function

Uric acid is an end product from the degradation of the purine nucleosides, adenosine and guanosine. In mammals, uricase breaks uric acid further down to allantoin which is then excreted in urine [1]. Humans lack this enzyme, leaving uric acid as the end product. This has led researchers to take a closer look at the function of uric acid. In 1981 one of the leading articles was published by Ames et el. in which they stated that have found evidence that uric acid has the ability to function as a powerful antioxidant by scavenging single oxygens and radicals and at physiological levels has further protective properties on erythrocytes that are comparable with ascorbate [2]. These findings about urate's antioxidative function were again confirmed in 2008 by Sautin and Johnson but the researchers added that uric acid can be pro-inflammatory through oxidative properties. Interestingly, they discovered that uric acid can have execute different effects in different parts of the body. In plasma, uric acid functions as an antioxidant and within cells as a pro-oxidant which led them to refer to this contradiction as the oxidant-antioxidant paradox [3]. This paradox explains that hyperuricemia can lead to an inflammatory response causing gout, endothelial dysfunction causing cardiovascular diseases [4] and it can act as a neuroprotector via the antioxidant capacity of uric acid and subsequent reduction of oxidative damage. On the other hand, low uric acid levels have been shown to decrease the activity of myeloperoxidase and increase lipid peroxidation through the loss of the antioxidant properties of uric acid [5]. The reduced antioxidant capacity is believed to be neurotoxic due to increased oxidative damage [6] but it remains unclear if this loss is sufficient to induce neurodegenerative diseases [7].

2.1 Mortality and serum uric acid levels

There has been a long history of research focusing on the effects of hyperuricemia and its clinical significance. If uric acid levels exceed the baseline the pro-oxidative effect causes damage to the tissue which can induce disease. As an example, hyperuricemia has been widely accepted as an independent risk factor for hypertension due to the inflammatory response by urate that can lead to endothelial dysfunction, however hyperuricemia remains controversial whether it is an independent risk factor for cardiovascular disease. In 2006, the Rotterdam study claimed that hyperuricemia is a risk factor for cardiovascular disease and stroke [8] while this claim was refuted in 2016 by Kuwabara who states that there are too many cofounders to establish this association [9]. Another pathology that has hyperuricemia as a risk factor, is gout. This inflammatory arthritis occurs when serum urate levels are saturated that monosodium urate crystals form and deposit in the joints leading to intense pain and discomfort. The most commonly prescribed treatment for gout prevention is urate lowering medication such as allopurinol while for acute flares non-steroidal anti-inflammatory drugs are used. When using urate lowering medication, the current guidelines and their respective uric acid levels become of interest. In the current European guidelines for the treatment of gout, it is recommended that uric acid levels should be less than 6 mg/dL but not less than 3 mg/dL [10]. It is noteworthy that the lower threshold has been established due to the lack of improvement for gout rather than the potential sequela of hypouricemia.

The mortality from high and from low uric acid has been investigated by several studies. One example is the EPOCH-Japan study which is a large-scale review of 13 cohort studies in Japan. The results showed that low uric acid levels have an increased overall mortality from cardiovascular diseases. They concluded a J- or U-shaped association between low and high uric acid levels and cardiovascular mortality [11]. Another study conducted in Korea also confirms a U-shaped, independent relationship between serum uric acid level and mortality [12]. The relationship between mortality and hyperuricemia can be explained by the activation of the NLRP3 inflammasome and a resulting increase of Interleukin-1ß and increased production of ROS [13] which then trigger arteriosclerosis [9]. However, how exactly hypouricemia is associated with mortality has not been fully understood as of now. Possible explanations given by the authors of the Korean study were malnutrition, side effects of medications that affect urate levels, other comorbidities, and increased risk of oxidative stress due to a reduction in the antioxidative properties of uric acid.

2.2 Causes of hypouricemia

The definition for hypouricemia is serum urate levels less than 2 mg/dL [14]. The causes can be either through inherited disorders that decrease the uric production such as hereditary xanthinuria or purine nucleosidase phosphorylase deficiency or disorders that increase the urinary excretion of urate such as inherited familial renal hypouricemia or acquired disorders such as Fanconi syndrome. More commonly, however, is hypouricemia through a secondary process such a urate lowering medication which are commonly used in the management of gout or uric acid oxidation with derivatives of uricase that are commonly used in oncology.

2.3 Inherited hypouricemia

To study the effects of hypouricemia, researchers have been focusing on patients with cases of inherited low uric acid. For these patients, it has been established that the low uric acid levels are not due to another disease or condition that influences serum uric acid level and therefore, patients with inherited low uric acid make an ideal model to study the possible risks of urate-lowering therapies without a lower threshold. In theory that sounds very promising, however inherited defects causing decreased uric acid production are very rare and often are incidental findings. Familial renal hypouricemia, a genetic condition causing increased excretion of uric acid through a loss of function mutation in the renal tubular urate transporter, is among the most commonly studied condition and while its prevalence worldwide is unknown, it has been established that it is more common in Asian countries such as Japan (prevalence: 0.3%) [15] and South Korea (prevalence: 1.39%) [16]. Two types of familial renal hypouricemia have been defined: for renal hypouricemia type 1 the mutation is in the SLC22A12 gene (URAT1 transporter) while the mutation for renal hypouricemia type 2 is in the SLC2A9 gene (GLUT9). Most commonly patients remain asymptomatic with these mutations, however both types have been linked to cases of nephrolithiasis and exercise-induced acute kidney injury (EIAKI) while renal hypouricemia type 2 has additionally been linked to a more severe condition, the posterior reversible encephalopathy syndrome (PRES), which presents with headache, seizures, and other neurological findings. In 2012, a case report by Fujinaga et al. was published in the European Journal of Pediatrics about a child with familial renal hypouricemia type 1 and PRES. In the case report they suggest that PRES is not due to severe hypouricemia per se, but rather an adverse effect of severe EIAKI [17]. For further understanding on how renal hypouricemia can cause posterior reversible encephalopathy syndrome more research is needed.

2.4 Acquired hypouricemia

By far the most common cause of acquired hypouricemia is due to the use of urate-lowering therapies and subsequent decreased uric acid production [18]. These therapies are most commonly used in the treatment of gout which is a disease characterized by abnormal uric acid crystal formation and deposition due to elevated plasma uric acid levels. Deposits of uric acid crystals are commonly referred to as a tophus or tophi. For the control of clinically significant gout flares, urate lowering therapy such as xanthine oxidase inhibitors and recombinant uricase or uricosuric agents are prescribed. Recombinant uricase and uricosuric agents are typically used in more severe cases. In most guidelines the recommendation is to lower plasma urate below 6 mg/dL. If tophi are present guidelines suggest to further lower plasma urate below 5 mg/dL [10, 19–23]. There are only two guidelines, the British Society for Rheumatology [20] and EULAR recommendation [10] that mention potential outcomes from lowering urate levels. It is believed that low urate levels increase the risk for neurodegenerative disorders [24] such as Parkinson's disease, Alzheimer's disease and Amyotrophic lateral sclerosis and elevated levels may have a protective function [6, 25]. Furthermore, in the past decade the results of seven randomized clinical trials have been published that investigated potential dangers of urate-lowering therapy by the three most commonly used therapies (Xanthine oxidase inhibitors, recombinant uricase and uricosuric agents) [26–32]. In the largest trial, the CARES study, a statistically significant relationship between intensive urate lowering therapy and mortality was found [32]. In the other trials this relationship was not statistically significant but mortality was highest in the arms with the greatest urate lowering effect, raising the suspicion of safety concerns with commonly used gout medication without a lower cut-off threshold [33]. To date only EULAR recommendations suggest a specific threshold, in this case not lower than 3 mg/dL. Other than EULAR and the British Society for Rheumatology [10, 20], no major published guidelines currently address the potential dangers of lowering urate levels beyond the normal range.

2.5 Adverse effects of hypouricemia

There is still little conclusive evidence about the specific short- and long-term clinical effects of hypouricemia, despite the fact that several research have shown a general relationship between mortality and both hyper- and hypouricemia. A theoretical concern as no cases (except for patients with tumor lysis syndrome) have been reported to date [34], is the possible risk from using urate-lowering medication with xanthine oxidase inhibitors that could lead to hypoxanthine and xanthine build up that then consequently could potentially cause xanthine nephropathy. Emerging research established that the physiologic function of normal serum uric acid acts as a protective antioxidant and the subsequent loss of this function when levels are below normal, however research has not been able to establish a definite relationship and only suspects a link between hypouricemia and the development of neurodegenerative disease.

3. Methodology

3.1 Study subjects

The following study was completed as an observational study in the period of September to December of 2019 at following four hospitals and clinics in Latvia: Daugavpils Regional Hospital, Orto Clinic, Riga East University Hospital and Pauls Stradins Clinical University Hospital. The patient selection was randomized of both inpatient and outpatient patients, whose serum uric acid was measured as part of their routine blood test. The criteria of exclusion were based on pathologies that could secondarily affect uric acid levels such as high creatinine and/or chronic kidney diseases, as well as patients receiving urate lowering medication and if the admission was related to a pathology directly affecting the patient's uric acid concentration. Lastly, patients who refused to allow their data to be used for research reasons were also not included in the study. Included patients were asked to sign a consent form and were interviewed regarding their age, height, weight and history of myocardial infarction or stroke (and at what age it occurred) and whether they have been diagnosed with a neurodegenerative disease. As a second step, the medical records were reviewed to confirm the patient's eligibility to be included in the research, as well as to confirm their medical history and information and to collect serum uric acid from the laboratory data. Lastly, the included patients were then stratified into two categories: patients with neurodegenerative disease and patients without neurodegenerative disease.

3.2 Variables

In accordance with the hospitals range of uric acid, hypouricemia was defined as less than 200 μmol/L and the most recent measurement of the routine blood testing was used for this research. Patients with elevated creatinine above 110 μmol/L were excluded from the study. Blood pressure measurements were performed once on the right arm. A large group of patients have had a history of hypertension and have been receiving anti-hypertensive treatment. The history of myocardial infarction or stroke was confirmed by review of the patient's medical chart. Neurodegenerative diseases of interest included Alzheimer's disease and vascular Dementia. Alzheimer's disease was defined as G30 in the ICD-10 classification and vascular Dementia was defined as F01.5 in ICD-10 classification. The ICD-10 classification have been translated from the Latvian SKK klasifikācija.

3.3 Statistical analysis

Statistical analysis was performed using statistical software SPSS (*Statistical package for the social sciences*, SPSS Inc., Chicago, IL), Version 20, 2018. Demographic data were expressed as mean with standard deviations. The statistical analysis was performed in accordance with objectives using following statistical methods: Kolmogorov-Smirnov test, Pearson correlation coefficient, two tailed t-test for independent means, Fisher exact probability test and chi-squared test. Statistical significance was set at $\alpha = 0.05$.

4. Results

4.1 Demographics

In total 100 patients were asked for their consent to participate in this study of which five declined and 18 patients were ineligible due to the exclusion criteria. The remaining 77 patients were stratified into two groups: 45 patients with a neurodegenerative disease and 32 patients without a neurodegenerative disease. The group of patients with neurodegenerative disease included 4 patients with Alzheimer's disease (G30 in ICD-10 classification), 40 patients with vascular dementia (F01.5 in ICD-10 classification) and one patient with a dementia in other disease classified elsewhere (F02.8 in ICD-10 classification). The average serum uric acid levels for patients with a neurodegenerative disease was 387 ± 210 μmol/L compared to 409 ± 156 μmol/L in patients without a neurodegenerative disease. There were six patients with a neurodegenerative disease whose serum uric acid levels fall below the normal range of 200 μmol/L. Further details of the study population are depicted in **Table 1**.

4.2 Uric acid correlation with age and kidney function

The kidneys, whose function decreases with age, excrete two-thirds of uric acid from the body [35, 36]. Therefore, the correlation between serum uric acid concentration and GFR was calculated. As expected, there is a moderate positive correlation ($r = 0.58$) for patients for neurodegenerative disease and ($r = 0.51$) demonstrated in **Figure 1** and for patients without this diagnosis demonstrated in **Figure 2**. Both results are statistically significant at $p < 0.05$. Additionally, the correlation between serum uric acid concentration and age in the subject of interest was tested by Pearson correlation coefficient. Results showed that in both groups there is a weak correlation ($r = 0.0615$) for patients with neurodegenerative diseases and ($r = -0.70$) for patients without neurodegenerative disease and both are statistically not significant at $p < 0.05$.

4.3 Uric acid differences between patients with neurodegenerative disease and patients without neurodegenerative disease

The selection of patients occurred randomly and were immediately stratified into the two groups of patients with neurodegenerative disease and without

Variables	Patients with neurodegenerative disease	Patients without neurodegenerative disease
Females	26	23
Males	19	9
Age in years	81 ± 10	70 ± 13
Weight in kg	75.6 ± 11	80.3 ± 14
Height in cm	170 ± 7	167 ± 9
BMI	26.3 ± 11	28.8 ± 13
Uric acid in μmol/L	387 ± 210	409 ± 156
Creatinine in μmol/L	83 ± 26	76 ± 20
GFR in mL/min/1.73 m^2	98 ± 16	96 ± 14
Alzheimer's disease patients	4	NA
Vascular dementia patients	40	NA
Dementia in other diseases classified elsewhere	1	NA
Systolic blood pressure in mmHg	131 ± 18	122 ± 12
Diastolic blood pressure in mmHg	74 ± 10	79 ± 8
Myocardial infarction patients	0	5 (average age 73)
Single stroke episode patients	3 (average age 71)	3 (average age 60)

Table 1.
Demographics of the study population.

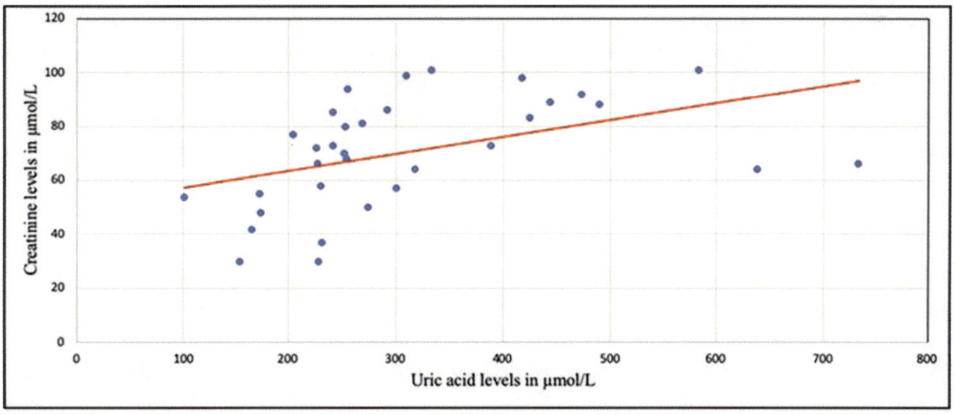

Figure 1.
Moderate positive correlation between uric acid levels and creatinine levels in patients with neurodegenerative disease.

neurodegenerative disease regardless of their uric acid levels. To investigate whether a difference of the uric acid levels exists between those two groups, a two tailed t-test for two independent means with a significance level $p < 0.05$ was used. The result was statistically not significant $t = -0.50$, $p = 0.62$, meaning that there is no difference in the uric acid concentrations within the two groups.

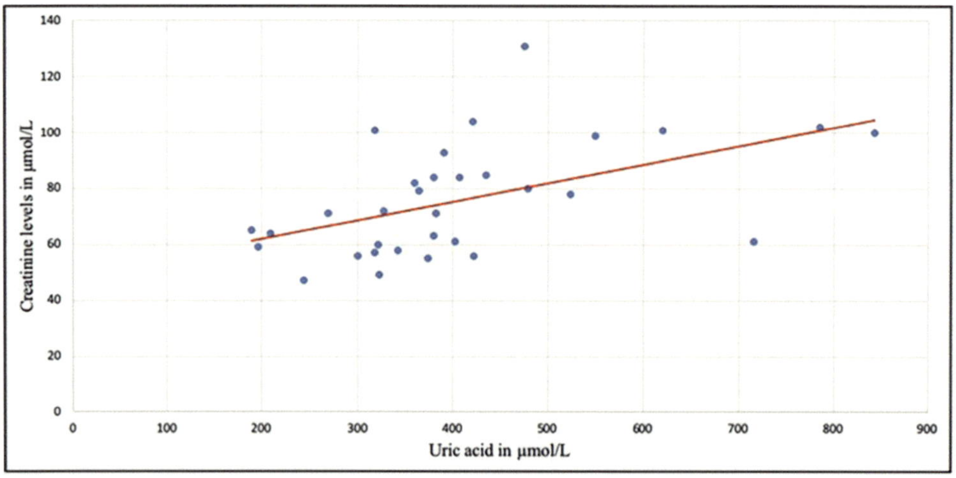

Figure 2.
Moderate positive correlation between uric acid levels and creatinine levels in patients without neurodegenerative disease.

4.4 Uric acid differences and its association with myocardial infarction and stroke

Whether hyperuricemia is a risk factor for cardiovascular has been controversial over the past decade and the most recent consensus was that there are too many confounders to claim hyperuricemia as an independent risk factor for cardiovascular disease. For the patient population in this research, the authors wanted to investigate whether there is a statistically significant association between serum uric acid levels and patient's history of myocardial infarcts and strokes. The stratified patient groups were tested for a statistically significant relationship between uric acid levels and myocardial infarction with a Fisher exact probability test. The result was statistically significant with a significance level $p < 0.05$. The same test was used to test for a statistically significant relationship between uric acid levels and stroke for which the result was statistically not significant $p = 0.69$. This means there is detectable association in both groups between uric acid levels in patients with myocardial infarction and patients without a myocardial infarction. However, this association cannot be found for patients with a single stroke episode.

4.5 Uric acid differences and its association with neurodegenerative diseases in stratified age groups

Both groups, the group of patients with a neurodegenerative disease and the group of patients without neurodegenerative disease, were then stratified into the age group 50–79 years and patients over the age of 80 due to the possible influence of increased age on vascular dementia. The average uric acid levels for the different age groups can be seen in **Figure 3**. The stratified group was tested with a Fisher exact probability test for a statistically significant relationship between the two age groups and the diagnosis of vascular dementia which was statistically significant with a significance level $p < 0.05$. If the same stratified group was tested for the statistically significant relationship of the age groups and Alzheimer's disease, the result was statistically not

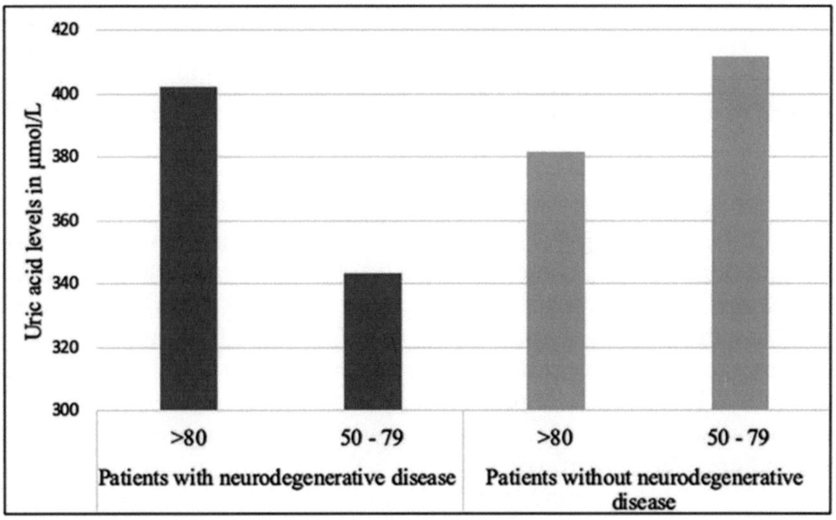

Figure 3.
Average uric acid levels in different age groups.

significant. Due to the statistically significant relationship between the stratified age groups and vascular dementia and the earlier result of our statistical analysis that showed a weak positive correlation between age and serum uric acid levels, the same stratified age groups were tested for their uric acid levels with a two tailed t-test for two independent means for a statistically significant difference. The result was not significant $t = -2.0$, $p = 0.07$.

4.6 Hypouricemia and its association with neurodegenerative diseases

The focus of interest of this study was the potential association between hypouricemia and neurodegenerative diseases. To investigate this potential relationship the first step was to explore how patients with hypouricemic levels compared to patients with normal uric acid levels for their rate in vascular dementia and for their rate in Alzheimer's disease. A chi-squared test of independence with a significance level $p < 0.05$ was used and showed a non-random association between the rate of vascular dementia in patients with hypouricemia and patients with normal serum uric acid levels. This finding was not statistically significant x^2 (1, N = 77) =0.56, $p = 0.45$ which indicates that there is no significant difference in the rate of vascular dementia regardless of the uric acid levels. The same test was used to investigate Alzheimer's disease and the results showed a non-random distribution that was statistically significant x^2 (1, N = 77) = 10.5, $p = 0.001$. Therefore, it can be concluded that there is a statistically significant difference of Alzheimer's disease in patients with hypouricemia and patients with normal uric acid.

5. Discussion

Uric acid has a complex function in the body. It can induce inflammation, endothelial dysfunction, and oxidative stress but it is also known to be a powerful antioxidant. This is known as the oxidant-antioxidant paradox. Laboratory studies have shown that the loss of uric acid causes a reduction in antioxidant capacity. This is mediated by decreased myeloperoxidase activity and increased lipid peroxidation and subsequent oxidative damage. Research has shown that this oxidative damage can be linked to neurodegenerative diseases such as Parkinson's disease and Multiple Sclerosis [37].

The pathogenesis of Alzheimer's disease is characterized primarily by the accumulation of neurotoxic metabolic products and abnormal proteins such a beta amyloid and neurofibrillary tangles [38, 39]. This creates an environment hostile to normal brain cell function and results in progressive dysregulation and synaptic dysfunction. Several studies have implicated neuronal excitotoxicity from overstimulation of N-methyl-D-aspartate (NMDA) receptors [40]. These specific neurotoxic processes may be counteracted by neuroprotective factors in the brain, with the antioxidative effects of normal blood uric acid playing a significant role. In patients with hypouricemia the loss of this neuroprotective effect could exacerbate damage from excitoxic pathways and unchecked neuronal loss.

However, vascular dementia has showed conflicting results in recent research and does not appear to be related to lower uric acid levels. This does not come as a surprise, given the large number of risk factors and the multifactorial etiologies of vascular dementia. Even while certain neuroprotective variables could contribute to the development or severity of vascular dementia, the relative importance of these factors may be overwhelmed by the greater effects of cardiovascular, renal, and overall endothelial risk factors.

The positive result for the chi-squared test of independence in the rate of Alzheimer's disease between patients with hypouricemia and patients with normal serum uric acid levels gives weight to the neuroprotective hypothesis of normal serum uric acid levels, and the possible effects of its loss in patients with hypouricemia. Similarly, the negative result of the chi-square analysis in patients with vascular dementia provides some reinforcement to the idea that the multiple risk factors of vascular dementia may outweigh any potential neuroprotective effects of normal uric acid levels. Another possibility is that uric acid may have no role in vascular dementia given a statistically not significant result of the t-test indicated there is no association between the means of uric acid in stratified age groups with vascular dementia. Furthermore, the results of the Fisher exact probability tests showed that age is a definitive influence on vascular dementia, but it had no effect on the rate of Alzheimer's disease. Overall, these findings are consistent with previously published data that has indicated a potential neuroprotective effect of normal uric acid levels.

Analysis of this data set showed several other findings. Patients with neurodegenerative diseases did not have statistically significant different uric acid levels than those without such a diagnosis, however the small sample size of patients makes it challenging to interpret this one data point. Furthermore, the statistically significant result of the Fisher exact probability test of serum uric acid levels in the two patient groups and the history of myocardial infarction can also be attributed to execution of this research. Although patients were chosen at random, a sizable portion came from cardiology wards, increasing the possibility that myocardial infarction patients would be included in this study. Additionally, there was no upper threshold of uric acid levels for the analyzed subjects therefore patients with elevated uric acid levels, which is a controversial risk factor for cardiovascular diseases, were included in this study.

Patients with a history of single episode stroke and patients without a stroke in the two stratified patient groups were tested with a Fisher exact probability test which showed non statistically significant results. This was predicted because there is a significant overlap between the risk variables for chronic vascular dementia and single episode strokes. With the abundance of confounding variables of cardiovascular, renal, and endothelial risk factors, it could be that the potential neuroprotective effects of normal uric acid levels are diminished. While it is beyond the scope of this paper, it raises the question about whether the proposed antioxidative effects of normal blood uric acid levels have different roles in different organ systems, or if the antioxidative role of uric acid is uniquely important in neurodegeneration or general brain function.

Creatinine and serum uric acid levels on the other hand showed a moderate positive correlation and reached statistical significance. This is unsurprising as uric acid levels and creatinine, and general renal function are closely related.

There are three main limitations in this study. First, the sample size with 77 patients was relatively small. The sample size was sufficient enough to determine statistical significance in the most important test, however by having a larger study pool, the detection of all statistically significant association could have been ensured. The second drawback was that uric acid levels were a single time measurement and were not followed over a period of time, therefore any transient changes in hypo- or hyperuricemic status cannot be excluded. While patients placed on uric acid lowering medications and patients with renal insufficiency were excluded from the study, and therefore it is unlikely that overall uric acid status would change significantly, it is possible that serial measurements of uric acid levels would more confidently sort patients into appropriate hypo- and hyperuricemic categories. And lastly, while test subjects were drawn from inpatient and outpatient settings, the majority were hospitalized patients who were admitted for some medical pathology. It is therefore not possible to surely exclude any contributing factors to our results and as in many studies, dealing with hospitalized patient populations, there is a possibility that results may vary by patient population.

In conclusion, this study provides evidence that hypouricemia has potential effects on health, specifically on the rate of neurodegenerative diseases such as Alzheimer's disease. The lack of a statistically significant association for vascular dementia lends additional evidence to the potential role of uric acid as a factor in diseases mediated by specific neurodegenerative processes as opposed to a general neuroprotective effect. While no research to date has found convincing evidence for a particular lower bound of normal blood uric acid levels, this research furthers the argument that one is needed. In the absence of specific evidence-based recommendations the EULAR guidelines of maintaining blood uric acid levels between 3 mg/dL to 6 mg/dL seem prudent. Future research should focus on identifying other pathological associations with low uric acid levels and also on determining a definite lower bound of normal serum uric levels.

6. Conclusion

In conclusion, this research supports the findings of other emerging studies that there is a possible link between hypouricemia and its effect on the brain and cognitive abilities and provides further evidence for hypouricemia potentially being a risk factor for neurodegenerative diseases like Alzheimer's disease. As expected, this study did not provide evidence an association between hypouricemia and vascular dementia and hence further strengthens the potential role of uric acid as a factor in diseases mediated by specific neurodegenerative processes as opposed to a general neuroprotective effect.

The most important finding of this study remains that there is a definite need for a lower threshold for normal serum uric acid levels, especially for patients who are receiving novel urate-lowering therapies. As of now no research has established strong support to define an optimal range for uric acid levels, however the EULAR recommendations to keep blood uric acid levels between 3 mg/dL and 6 mg/dL seem appropriate in the absence of explicit evidence-based recommendations.

Conflict of interest

The authors declare no conflict of interest.

Author details

Anna Mihailova[1*†], Maximiliane Trapp[1†] and Natalija Kakurina[2]

1 Faculty of Medicine, Riga Stradins University, Riga, Latvia

2 Daugavpils University, Daugavpils, Latvia

*Address all correspondence to: annamihailova@inbox.lv

† These authors contributed equally.

References

[1] Maiuolo J, Oppedisano F, Gratteri S, Muscoli C, Mollace V. Regulation of uric acid metabolism and excretion. International Journal of Cardiology. 2016;**213**:8-14. DOI: 10.1016/j.ijcard.2015.08.109

[2] Ames BN, Cathcart R, Schwiers E, Hochstein P. Uric acid provides an antioxidant defense in humans against oxidant- and radical-caused aging and cancer: A hypothesis. Proceedings of the National Academy of Sciences. 1981;**78**(11):6858-6862. DOI: 10.1073/pnas.78.11.6858

[3] Sautin YY, Johnson RJ. Uric acid: The oxidant-antioxidant paradox. Nucleosides, Nucleotides & Nucleic Acids. 2008;**27**(6):608-619. DOI: 10.1080/15257770802138558

[4] Kanbay M, Segal M, Afsar B, Kang D-H, Rodriguez-Iturbe B, Johnson RJ. The role of uric acid in the pathogenesis of human cardiovascular disease. Heart. 2013;**99**(11):759-766. DOI: 10.1136/heartjnl-2012-302535

[5] Becker BD, Coremans C, Chaumont M, Delporte C, Antwerpen PV, Franck T, et al. Severe hypouricemia impairs endothelium-dependent vasodilatation and reduces blood pressure in healthy young men: A randomized, placebo-controlled, and crossover study. Journal of the American Heart Association. 2019;**8**(23):5-10. DOI: 10.1161/jaha.119.013130

[6] Luo XLJJ. A double-edged sword: Uric acid and neurological disorders. Brain Disorders & Therapy. 2013;**02**(02):3-4. DOI: 10.4172/2168-975x.1000109

[7] Settle T, Klandorf H. The role of uric acid as an antioxidant in selected neurodegenerative disease pathogenesis: A short review. Brain Disorders & Therapy. 2014;**03**(03):2-5. DOI: 10.4172/2168-975x.1000129

[8] Bos MJ, Koudstaal PJ, Hofman A, Witteman JCM, Breteler MMB. Uric acid is a risk factor for myocardial infarction and stroke. Stroke. 2006;**37**(6):1503-1507

[9] Kuwabara M. Hyperuricemia, cardiovascular disease, and hypertension. Pulse. 2016;**3**(3-4):242-252. DOI: 10.1159/000443769

[10] Richette P, Doherty M, Pascual E, et al. 2016 updated EULAR evidence-based recommendations for the management of gout. Annals of the Rheumatic Diseases. 2017;**76**:29-42. Available from: https://ard.bmj.com/content/76/1/29

[11] Zhang W, Iso H, Murakami Y, Miura K, Nagai M, Sugiyama D, et al. Serum uric acid and mortality form cardiovascular disease: EPOCH-JAPAN study. Journal of Atherosclerosis and Thrombosis. 2016;**23**(6):692-703. DOI: 10.5551/jat.31591

[12] Cho SK, Chang Y, Kim I, Ryu S. U-shaped association between serum uric acid level and risk of mortality. Arthritis & Rheumatology. 2018;**70**(7):1122-1132. DOI: 10.1002/art.40472

[13] Braga TT, Forni MF, Correa-Costa M, Ramos RN, Barbuto JA, Branco P, et al. Soluble uric acid activates the NLRP3 Inflammasome. Scientific Reports. 2017;**7**(1):2-9. DOI: 10.1038/srep39884

[14] Esparza Martin N, Garcia NV. Hypouricemia and tubular transport of uric acid. Nefrología. 2011;**31**:44-50

[15] Nakayama A, Matsuo H, Ohtahara A, Ogino K, Hakoda M, Hamada T, et al.

Clinical practice guideline for renal hypouricemia (1st edition). Human Cell. 2019;**32**(2):83-87. DOI: 10.1007/s13577-019-00239-3

[16] Son C-N, Kim J-M, Kim S-H, Cho S-K, Choi C-B, Sung Y-K, et al. Prevalence and possible causes of hypouricemia at a tertiary care hospital. The Korean Journal of Internal Medicine. 2016;**31**(5):971-976. DOI: 10.3904/kjim.2015.125

[17] Fujinaga S, Ito A, Nakagawa M, Watanabe T, Ohtomo Y, Shimizu T. Posterior reversible encephalopathy syndrome with exercise-induced acute kidney injury in renal hypouricemia type 1. European Journal of Pediatrics. 2013;**172**(11):1557-1560. DOI: 10.1007/s00431-013-1986-7

[18] Mount DB, Sterns RH, Forman JP. Hypouricemia: Causes and clinical significance. In: Post TW, editor. UpToDate. Waltham, MA: UpToDate; 2018. Available from https://www.uptodate.com/contents/hypouricemia-causes-and-clinical-significance

[19] Yu K-H, Chen D-Y, Chen J-H, Chen S-Y, Chen S-M, Cheng T-T, et al. Management of gout and hyperuricemia: Multidisciplinary consensus in Taiwan. International Journal of Rheumatic Diseases. 2018;**21**(4):772-787. DOI: 10.1111/1756-185x.13266

[20] Hui M, Carr A, Cameron S, Davenport G, Doherty M, Forrester H, et al. The British society for rheumatology guideline for the management of gout. Rheumatology. 2017;**56**(7):e1-e20. DOI: 10.1093/rheumatology/kex156

[21] Kiltz U, Alten R, Fleck M, Krüger K, Manger B, Müller-Ladner U, et al. Evidenzbasierte Empfehlung zur Diagnostik und Therapie der Gichtarthritis im fachärztlichen Sektor. Zeitschrift für Rheumatologie. 2017;**76**(2):118-124. DOI: 10.1007/s00393-016-0249-1

[22] Sautner J, Gruber J, Herold M, Zwerina J, Leeb BF. Österreichische 3e-Empfehlungen zu Diagnose und Management von Gicht 2013. Wiener Klinische Wochenschrift. 2013;**126**(3-4):79-89. DOI: 10.1007/s00508-013-0469-1

[23] Graf SW, Whittle SL, Wechalekar MD, Moi JHY, Barrett C, Hill CL, et al. Australian and New Zealand recommendations for the diagnosis and management of gout: Integrating systematic literature review and expert opinion in the 3e initiative. International Journal of Rheumatic Diseases. 2015;**18**(3):341-351. DOI: 10.1111/1756-185x.12557

[24] Bowman GL, Shannon J, Frei B, Kaye JA, Quinn JF. Uric acid as a CNS antioxidant. Journal of Alzheimers Disease. 2010;**19**(4):1331-1336. DOI: 10.3233/jad-2010-1330

[25] Paganoni S, Schwarzschild MA. Urate as a marker of risk and progression of neurodegenerative disease. Neurotherapeutics. 2016;**14**(1):148-153. DOI: 10.1007/s13311-016-0497-4

[26] Sundy JS, Baraf HSB, Yood RA, et al. Efficacy and tolerability of Pegloticase for the treatment of chronic gout in patients refractory to conventional treatment: Two randomized controlled trials. JAMA. 2011;**306**(7):711-720. DOI: 10.1001/jama.2011.1169

[27] Tausche A-K, Alten R, Dalbeth N, Kopicko J, Fung M, Adler S, et al. Lesinurad monotherapy in gout patients intolerant to a xanthine oxidase inhibitor: A 6 month phase 3 clinical

trial and extension study. Rheumatology. 2017;**56**(12):2170-2178. DOI: 10.1093/rheumatology/kex350

[28] Dalbeth N, Jones G, Terkeltaub R, Khanna D, Kopicko J, Bhakta N, et al. Lesinurad, a selective uric acid reabsorption inhibitor, in combination with Febuxostat in patients with Tophaceous gout: Findings of a phase III clinical trial. Arthritis & Rheumatology. 2017;**69**(9):1903-1913. DOI: 10.1002/art.40159

[29] Saag KG, Fitz-Patrick D, Kopicko J, Fung M, Bhakta N, Adler S, et al. Lesinurad combined with allopurinol: A randomized, double-blind, placebo-controlled study in gout patients with an inadequate response to standard-of-care allopurinol (a US-based study). Arthritis & Rheumatology. 2016;**69**(1):203-212. DOI: 10.1002/art.39840

[30] Bardin T, Keenan RT, Khanna PP, et al. Lesinurad in combination with allopurinol: A randomised, double-blind, placebo-controlled study in patients with gout with inadequate response to standard of care (the multinational CLEAR 2 study). Annals of the Rheumatic Diseases. 2017;**76**:811-820

[31] Becker MA, Schumacher HR, Wortmann RL, Macdonald PA, Eustace D, Palo WA, et al. Febuxostat compared with allopurinol in patients with hyperuricemia and gout. New England Journal of Medicine. 2005;**353**(23):2450-2461. DOI: 10.1056/nejmoa050373

[32] White WB, Saag KG, Becker MA, Borer JS, Gorelick PB, Whelton A, et al. Cardiovascular safety of febuxostat or allopurinol in patients with gout. New England Journal of Medicine. 2018;**378**(13):1200-1210. DOI: 10.1056/nejmoa1710895

[33] Perez-Gomez MV, Bartsch L-A, Castillo-Rodriguez E, Fernandez-Prado R, Kanbay M, Ortiz A. Potential dangers of serum urate-lowering therapy. The American Journal of Medicine. 2019;**132**(4):457-467. DOI: 10.1016/j.amjmed.2018.12.010

[34] Bellomo G, Selvi A. Uric acid: The lower the better? Contributions to Nephrology Uric Acid in Chronic Kidney Disease. 2018;**192**:69-76. DOI: 10.1159/000484280

[35] Weinstein JR, Anderson S. The aging kidney: Physiological changes. Advances in Chronic Kidney Disease. 2010;**17**(4):302-307. DOI: 10.1053/j.ackd.2010.05.002

[36] Jalal DI. Hyperuricemia, the kidneys, and the spectrum of associated diseases: A narrative review. Current Medical Research and Opinion. 2016;**32**(11):1863-1869. DOI: 10.1080/03007995.2016.1218840

[37] Singh J. Gout and neurological disease: Is there a link?. Poster presented at: Annual American College of Rheumatology (ACR). Atlanta, GA. 11 Nov 2019

[38] Kocahan S, Doğan Z. Mechanisms of Alzheimer's disease pathogenesis and prevention: The brain, neural pathology, N-methyl-D-aspartate receptors, tau protein and other risk factors. Clinical Psychopharmacology and Neuroscience: The Official Scientific Journal of the Korean College of Neuropsychopharmacology. 2017;**15**(1):1-8. DOI: 10.9758/cpn.2017.15.1.1

[39] Longo FM, Massa SM. Neuroprotective strategies in Alzheimer's disease. NeuroRx : the Journal of the American Society for Experimental NeuroTherapeutics. 2004;**1**(1):117-127. DOI: 10.1602/neurorx.1.1.117

[40] Olivares D, Deshpande VK, Shi Y, Lahiri DK, Greig NH, Rogers JT, et al. N-methyl D-aspartate (NMDA) receptor antagonists and Memantine treatment for Alzheimer's disease, vascular dementia and Parkinson's disease. Current Alzheimer Research. 2012;**9**(6):746-758. DOI: 10.2174/156720512801322564

Chapter 7

Mixed Adenoneuroendocrine Carcinoma in the Colon: A Case Report

Murat Can Mollaoğlu

Abstract

Tumors that have both neuroendocrine and exocrine components in the gastrointestinal system are rare. One of the rarest places in the gastrointestinal system is the colon. These tumors are called mixed adenoneuroendocrine carcinomas (MANEC). To diagnose MANEC, the neuroendocrine and exocrine components that make up the lesion must be present at least 30%. A 70-year-old female patient with complaints of abdominal distension, malnutrition, nausea, and vomiting was admitted to our clinic from another center. The patient underwent blood tests, whole abdominal tomography, and colonoscopy. Right hemicolectomy and retroperitoneal lymph node dissection were performed with the preliminary diagnosis of colon cancer. Histopathological diagnosis was MANEC, and tumor stage was T3N1M0. Adjuvant chemotherapy was applied. Although MANEC is rare, it is a difficult and complex cancer to diagnose due to its nonspecific features. Diagnosis is made with histopathological and immunohistochemical evaluation along with clinical suspicion. Treatment is surgery and adjuvant therapy.

Keywords: adenocarcinoma, adenoneuroendocrine carcinoma, mixed adenoneuroendocrine carcinomas, neuroendocrine tumor, colon cancer

1. Introduction

Colon adenocarcinomas are the most common malignancy of the gastrointestinal tract, and the frequency of cancer development according to their histological types is 2–3% in tubular adenoma, 6–8% in tubulovillous adenoma, and 29–70% in villous adenoma [1]. Colon adenocarcinomas are the most common cancer of the digestive system and more than 50% of them progress with metastasis. Ki-67: It is an antigen that responds to nuclear nonhistone protein expressed in G1, G2, M, and S proliferative phases, and there is generally a good correlation between mitotic number and Ki-67. It is associated with cell proliferation [2]. Mixed adenoneuroendocrine carcinoma (MANEC) includes neoplasms that contain both neuroendocrine carcinomatous and adenocarcinomatous components. Its morphology is similar to that of advanced adenocarcinoma and differs from neuroendocrine tumors (G1 or G2), which usually present as a submucosal tumor with or without delle [1–3].

The neuroendocrine system includes endocrine glands such as the pituitary, parathyroid, and neuroendocrine adrenal. Endocrine islet tissues are found scattered within the exocrine parenchyma, such as the digestive and respiratory systems, as well as within the thyroid and pancreas. The gastrointestinal tract is the region where neuroendocrine cells are commonly located and 2/3 of neuroendocrine tumors (NETs) are located [4]. Neuroendocrine tumors (NET) are a heterogeneous group of tumors originating from neuroendocrine cells. These cells are specialized cells that have the ability to produce, store and secrete peptides, and biogenic amines. The common feature of these tumors is that they express both neural and endocrine markers, so they are called gastroenteropancreatic neuroendocrine tumor (GEP-NET). NETs are divided into two main groups: well-differentiated neuroendocrine tumor and poorly differentiated neuroendocrine carcinoma. Well-differentiated neuroendocrine tumors are called carcinoid tumors. Neuroendocrine tumors have been described in the central nervous system, respiratory system, larynx, gastrointestinal (GI) tract, thyroid, skin, breast, and urogenital tract [3, 5].

According to the WHO 2010 classification of GEP-NETs (**Table 1**), it provides a grading and naming system based on the morphological characteristics of tumors and cell proliferation rates, according to the criteria put forward by the European Neuroendocrine Tumor Society (ENETS) [6]. The common feature of these tumors is that they express both neural and endocrine markers, so they are called gastroentero-pancreatic neuroendocrine tumor.

In 2019, common classification criteria for all NETs were republished by WHO (**Table 1**). The main feature of this new classification is to distinguish well-differentiated neuroendocrine tumor, previously known as carcinoid tumor of the gastrointestinal tract, from poorly differentiated neuroendocrine carcinoma. In general, distinguishing between well-differentiated and slow-growing neuroendocrine neoplasms and poorly differentiated and fast-growing neuroendocrine neoplasms is of great clinical importance. The two main groups, which are primarily divided into poorly differentiated and well-differentiated neuroendocrine neoplasms according to histomorphologic features, actually differ from each other genetically, molecularly, biologically and morphologically except for neuroendocrine features. Neuroendocrine neoplasms are evaluated morphologically and grouped as neuroendocrine tumor (NET) and neuroendocrine carcinoma (NEC) according to the degree of differentiation into the cells from which they originate. This distinction is supported by genetic evidence, and it is known that tumors differ clinically and prognostically [5–7, 9–12].

Although colon NETs are rare, rectal NETs constitute 20% of GEP-NETs. It is seen in 5–6 Decade, and the incidence is equal in men and women. Colon NETs are histologically poorly differentiated neuroendocrine carcinoma. Metastasis is usually present at the time of diagnosis. It has a severe prognosis. Abdominal pain and weight loss may occur. Carcinoid syndrome may develop in less than 5% of patients. Rectal NETs are more common and have a better prognosis than colonic ones [12, 13]. They are mostly asymptomatic, and carcinoid syndrome is not observed. Patients with symptoms usually present with rectal bleeding, pain, or constipation. Most are smaller than 1 cm. Metastases can be seen in tumors larger than 2 cm and with invasion of the muscularis propria. Poorly differentiated neuroendocrine carcinomas have a poor prognosis. All neuroendocrine carcinomas are high-grade carcinomas. They show neuroendocrine differentiation both morphologically and immunohistochemically. Morphologically, they are divided into two groups: small cell and large cell. In the small cell group, cells have fine granular chromatin, and narrow cytoplasm and show morphological features, such as nuclear molding. In the large cell group,

WHO 1980	WHO 2000	WHO 2010	2019
• Carcinoid	• Well-differentiated neuroendocrine tumor • Well-differentiated neuroendocrine carcinoma • Poorly differentiated neuroendocrine carcinoma / small cell carcinoma	• Neuroendocrine tumor (NET) G1 • Neuroendocrine tumor (NET) G2 • Neuroendocrine carcinoma (NEC) (large cell or small cell type)	• Neuroendocrine tumor (NET) G1 • Neuroendocrine tumor (NET) G2 • Neuroendocrine tumor (NET) G3 • Neuroendocrine carcinoma (NEC) G3 (large or small cell type)
• Mucocarcinoid • Carcinoid-adenocarcinoma mixed forms • Pseudotumor lesions	• Mixed exocrine-endocrine carcinoma	• Mixed adenoneuroendocrine carcinoma (MANEC)	• Mixed neuroendocrine non-carcinoid- (MANEK) neuroendocrine neoplasia (MINEN)
• Pseudotumor lesions	• Tumor-like lesions	• Hyperplastic and preneoplastic lesions	

Table 1.
Classification of neuroendocrine tumors in the gastrointestinal system [6–8].

the cells have a moderate amount of cytoplasm and a round nucleus, sometimes with prominent nucleoli. NECs are aggressive tumors with high proliferative activity. The Ki67 proliferation index of tumors in this group is 20% and above. Most of the time it is above 75%. It is possible to see the Ki67 proliferation index around 20–50%, especially in cases exposed to chemotherapy. This is one of the situations confirming that the Ki67 index should not be used to differentiate neuroendocrine carcinomas and G3 neuroendocrine tumors [12–14].

Neuroendocrine tumors are rare in the colon and rectum, accounting for less than 2.0% of all colorectal malignancies. In some cases, neuroendocrine carcinoma and adenocarcinoma may occur together in the same tumor. According to the current classification of the World Health Organization (WHO), tumors in which neuroendocrine carcinoma and adenocarcinoma coexist are called "mixed adenoneuroendocrine carcinomas" (MANEC) [15]. MANEC is a neoplasm characterized by significant histological heterogeneity. In diagnosis, both neuroendocrine and adenocarcinoma components must be present simultaneously in ≥30% of cases. Mixed adenoneuroendocrine carcinoma, newly included in the 2010 WHO classification, is a rare tumor of the gastrointestinal tract that contains at least 30% of both adenocarcinoma and neuroendocrine carcinoma components. A total of 87% originates from the appendix. It is a very rare tumor in the colon and other parts of the gastrointestinal tract [1, 6, 15].

MANEC can be seen in every part of the gastrointestinal tract. The most common sites for MANEC are the esophagus [16], stomach [17, 18], appendix [19], gallbladder [20, 21], and pancreas [22]. It is rarely seen outside these regions. Although rare, cases of MANEC have been reported in areas, such as the colon [23–28] and duodenum [29]. The most common site of MANEC in the colon is the right colon (56%), followed by the left colon and transverse colon [27]. Colon NETs are usually EC cell NETs, while rectal NETs are usually L-cell NETs. Colon NETs form larger masses than NETs seen in other parts of the gastrointestinal tract. Rectal NETs are observed as small polyps or submucosal nodules. Most of these are in the G1 category [8, 27–29]. In this study, we present a rare case of MANEC that occurred in the ascending colon and was indistinguishable from adenocarcinoma.

2. Case report

A 70-year-old female patient with complaints of abdominal distension, malnutrition, nausea, and vomiting was admitted to our clinic from another center. Her clinical condition started 1 month ago and gradually worsened despite all conservative treatments. A mass was detected in the cecal region during the patient's colonoscopy. No malignancy was found in the biopsies. In the entire abdominal tomography performed in our center, there was wall thickening starting from the cecum and extending to the ascending colon, but no other pathology was found. Colonoscopy was tried twice, but could not be reached distal to the mass. No abnormality was detected in the initial laboratory values. The patient underwent emergency laparotomy. There was a 2×3×2 cm mass, obstructing the lumen in the transverse colon. The patient underwent extended right hemicolectomy and retroperitoneal lymph node dissection (**Figure 1**).

In the pathological examination of the sample, it was determined that there was adenocarcinoma 60% classical acinar and mucinous pattern + neuroendocrine carcinoma and 40% large cell type (**Figures 2** and **3**).

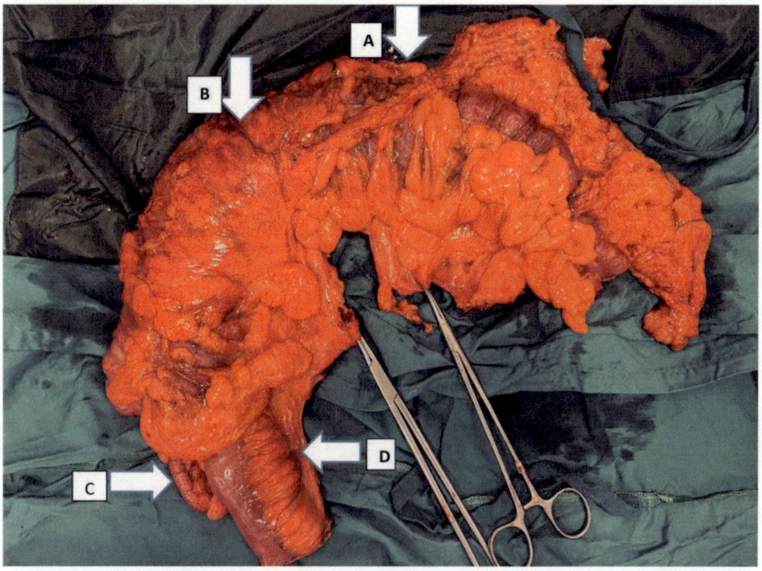

Figure 1.
Right hemicolectomy material A: Tumor B: Colon C: Appendix D: Ileum.

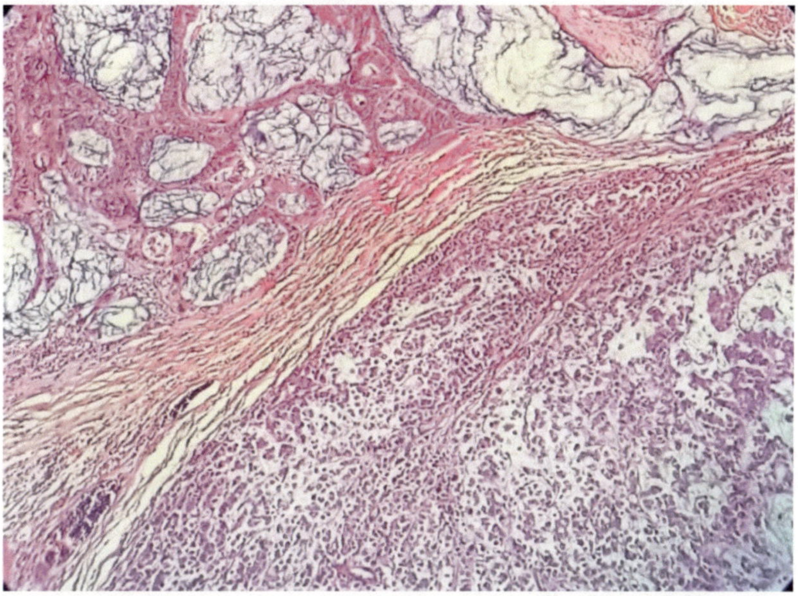

Figure 2.
Adenocarcinoma.

The tumor invaded the subserosal fat tissue (T3). The tumor was grade 3 (poorly differentiated) ulcerovegetan. A total of 25 lymph nodes were evaluated. There was reactive hyperplasia in 23 nodes and signs of carcinoma metastasis in two nodes (N1). Since the neuroendocrine component constituted a large part of the tumor, the pathologist had no difficulty in seeing it. Tumor markers, such as CEA, CA125, and CA19-9, were at normal levels. Distal and proximal surgical margins appeared

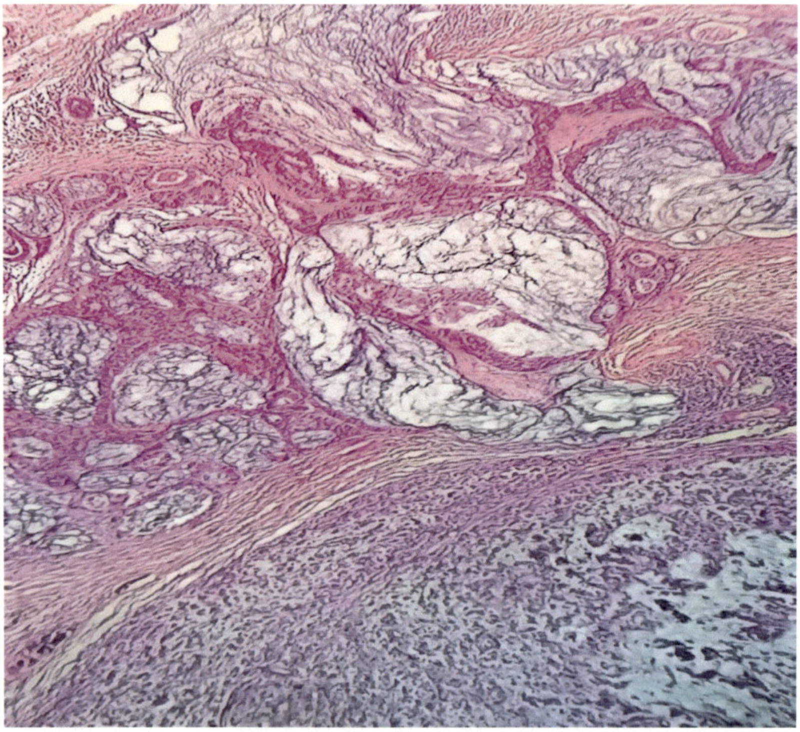

Figure 3.
Neuroendocrine tumor.

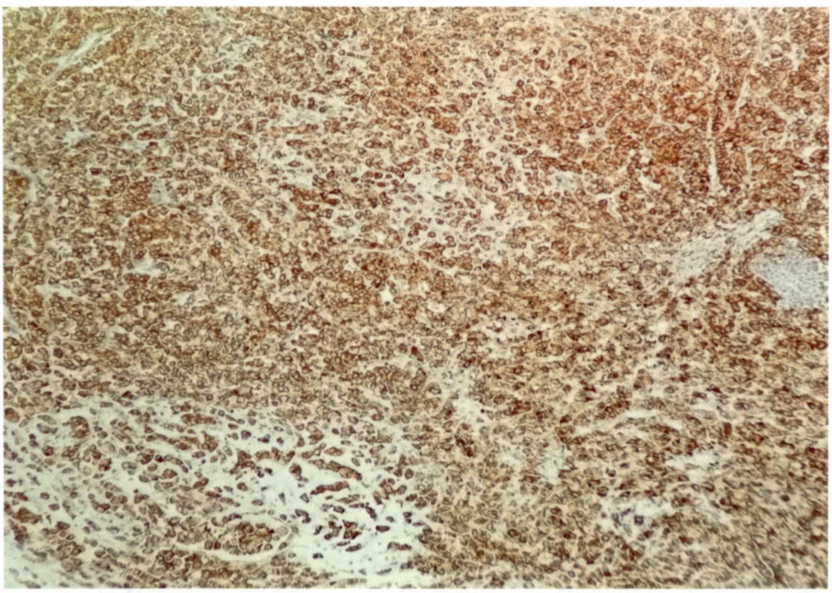

Figure 4.
Synaptophysin, immunohistochemical marker.

intact. Carcinoid syndrome was not observed in the patient. In immunohistochemical examination, there was diffuse staining with neuroendocrine component CD56 and synaptophysin (**Figure 4**). MLH6, MSH2, MSH6, and PMS were examined by immunohistochemical method and microsatellite instability was stable.

Ki-67 and synaptophysin are neuroendocrine-specific markers. They were also strongly stained in our patient [16, 27]. Ki-67 proliferation index was 80%. Histopathological stage was evaluated as T3N1bM0. Although Ki-67 was 80% and cisplatin (platinum) was suitable, treatment was started with etoposide because the general condition was poor, the ECOG performance score was two, and the creatinine level was at the border. Platinum-based treatment was not considered at the first stage. It was planned that platinum could be started depending on tolerance. The patient was given four cycles of etoposide. After the treatment was completed, the patient was evaluated with full abdominal CT and PET CT. During the period when this study was carried out on the case, the general condition of the patient tended to improve. No tumor deposits were found in control radiological examinations (abdomen CT, pet CT).

3. Discussion

MANEC is a rare tumor in the colorectal region. Therefore, studies on this tumor are limited. There are also a limited number of studies, although they are mostly in the form of case reports. Although the limited number of studies prevents us from drawing general conclusions regarding this tumor, the prognosis of these patients is worse than that of patients with routine colorectal cancer [30].

The definitive way to diagnose MANEC is through histopathological examination. How patients with MANEC will be treated, or how this disease will be managed has not been fully determined due to the rarity of these tumors. Treatment is usually directed at the more aggressive tumor component. Mixed adenoneuroendocrine carcinomas, containing a well-differentiated neuroendocrine tumor component and an adenocarcinoma component, should be treated as adenocarcinomas. Mixed adenoneuroendocrine carcinomas, containing a poorly differentiated neuroendocrine carcinoma component, should be considered as neuroendocrine carcinomas and treated accordingly [31]. The case we presented was also considered as neuroendocrine carcinoma and treated accordingly.

Some studies have shown that adjuvant chemotherapy is an effective treatment option for patients with MANEC [32]. However, it is not yet clear which chemotherapy regimen is most effective in treating patients with MANEC due to limited studies. Therefore, it is currently impossible to talk about the most effective chemotherapy regimen for patients with MANEC.

The clinical course of MANEC is neither similar to neuroendocrine carcinoma nor adenocarcinoma but different from both [33]. It is difficult to diagnose MANEC in these tumors without histopathological diagnosis. It does not have a specific clinical course or finding. Therefore, they are usually found by chance [2]. MANEC is usually diagnosed at an advanced stage, so its course is aggressive. Endoscopically, it appears as a semicircular or fungal tumor, covering the lumen with deep ulceration. However, due to their structural similarities, it is often difficult to differentiate from colorectal adenocarcinoma based on endoscopic appearance alone [33]. For this reason, like every colorectal tumor detected, histopathological examination and immunohistochemical staining are the most valuable diagnostic methods for MANEC, and for this, biopsy is required [2]. The National Comprehensive Cancer

Network (NCCN) recommends CT and MRI with intravenous contrast for clinical staging. Contrast-enhanced thoracoabdominopelvic CT is recommended for distant metastasis screening [34]. Although the sensitivity of F-fluorodeoxyglucose positron emission tomography for detecting nodal involvement in neuroendocrine tumors is high, its sensitivity in colorectal adenocarcinoma and neuroendocrine tumors is considered low at 42.9% and 33%, respectively [33]. Colonoscopy and abdominal CT were performed for the diagnosis and staging of the patient we presented.

4. Conclusion

In conclusion, MANEC is a malignant tumor prone to distant metastases. Therefore, diagnosis is usually made in the late and metastatic stage. Although more is known about its clinicopathological features today, a consensus has not been reached regarding both its clinicopathological features and its treatment. Our patient's clinical features and pathological features such as tumor localization, Ki-67, and tumor size were compatible with the literature. MANEC is a rare but highly aggressive disease. In this study, we aimed to present a rare colon MANEC patient to emphasize the term MANEC and to better understand the diagnosis, treatment, and management of MANEC. If the diagnosis is made in the early stages, surgical resection can be curative, but studies with a large number of patients are needed for the most appropriate treatment approach. More studies are needed to more clearly define how to manage patients with MANEC.

Author details

Murat Can Mollaoğlu
İstinye University, Gaziosmanpaşa Hospital, General Surgery Clinic, Istanbul, Turkey

*Address all correspondence to: mukaddermollaoglu@hotmail.com

References

[1] Dulskas A, Pilvelis A. Oncologic outcome of mixed adenoneuroendocrine carcinoma (MANEC): A single center case series. European Journal of Surgical Oncology. 2020;**46**(1):105-107

[2] Gonzalez HH, Skrove JL, Sharma R, Sobrado J. A rare case of mixed adenoneuroendocrine carcinoma of the ileocecal valve. Cureus. 2019;**11**:e3942

[3] Brathwaite S, Rock J, Yearsley MM, Bekaii-Saab T, Wei L, Frankel WL, et al. Mixed adeno-neuroendocrine carcinoma: An aggressive clinical entity. Annals of Surgical Oncology. 2016;**23**:2281e6

[4] Jiang M, Tan Y, Li X, Fu J, Hu H, Ye X, et al. Clinicopathological features and prognostic factors of colorectal neuroendocrine neoplasms. Gastroenterology Research and Practice. 2017;**2017**:4206172

[5] Kaltsas GA, Besser GM, Grossman AB. The diagnosis and medical management of advanced neuroendocrine tumors. Endocrine Reviews. 2004;**25**(3):458-511

[6] Bosman FT, World Health Organization, International Agency for Research on Cancer. WHO Classification of Tumours of the Digestive System. 4th ed. Lyon: International Agency for Research on Cancer; 2010

[7] Aydın HA. Gastrointestinal Kanal Nöroendokrin Tümörlerinin Histopatolojisi ve Güncel Tanısal Yaklaşım (Histopathology of gastrointestinal tract neuroendocrine tumors and current diagnostic approach). Güncel Gastroenteroloji Dergisi. 2023;**25**(1):26-36

[8] WHO Classification of Tumours Editorial Board. WHO Classification of Tumours of the Digestive System. 5th ed. Lyon: IARC Press; 2019

[9] Nagtegaal ID, Odze RD, Klimstra D, et al. The 2019 WHO classification of tumours of the digestive system. Histopathology. 2020;**76**:182-188

[10] Staren ED, Gould VE, Warren WH, Wool NL, Bines S, Baker J, et al. Neuroendocrine carcinomas of the colon and rectum: A clinicopathologic evaluation. Surgery. 1988;**104**:1080-1089

[11] Jesinghaus M, Konukiewitz B, Keller G, et al. Colorectal mixed adenoneuroendocrine carcinomas and neuroendocrine carcinomas are genetically closely related to colorectal adenocarcinomas. Modern Pathology. 2017;**30**:610-619

[12] Telli TA. Gastroenteropankreatik Nöroendokrin Tümörlerin Klinikopatolojik Özelliklerinin İncelenmesi. Ankara: Hacettepe Üniversitesi Tip Fakültesi İç Hastaliklari Anabilim Dali Uzmanlık Tezi; 2014

[13] Hamilton SR, Aaltonen LA, editors. WHO Classification of Tumours. Pathology and Genetics of Tumours of the Digestive System. Lyon: IARC Press; 2000

[14] Grabowski P, Schönfelder J, Ahnert Hilger G, et al. Expression of neuroendocrine markers: A signature of human undifferantiated carcinoma of the colon and rectum. Virchows Archiv. 2002;**441**:256-263

[15] Rindi G, Arnold R, Bosman FT. Nomenclature and classification of neuroendocrine neoplasms of the digestive system. In: Bosman FT, Carneiro F, Hruban RH, Theise ND,

et al., editors. WHO Classification of Tumors of the Digestive System. Lyon: IARC Press; 2010. pp. 13-14

[16] Kadhim MMK, Jespersen ML, Pilegaard HK, et al. Mixed adenoneuroendocrine carcinoma is a rare but important tumour found in the oesophagus. Case Reports in Gastrointestinal Medicine. 2016;**2016**:9542687

[17] Yamauchi H, Sakurai S, Nakazawa N, et al. A case of mixed adenoneuroendocrine carcinoma of the stomach with focal intestinal metaplasia and hypergastrinemia. International Surgery. 2015;**100**(3):562-567

[18] Kwok CM. Mixed adenoneuroendocrine carcinoma of the stomach. Case Reports in Gastroenterology. 2015;**9**(2):241-245

[19] Romeo M, Quer A, Tarrats A, Molina C, et al. Appendiceal mixed adenoneuroendocrine carcinomas, a rare entity that can present as a Krukenberg tumor: Case report and review of the literature. World Journal of Surgical Oncology. 2015;**13**:325

[20] Chen H, Shen YY, Ni XZ. Two cases of neuroendocrine carcinoma of the gallbladder. World Journal of Gastroenterology. 2014;**20**(33):11916-11920

[21] Lin ẎX, Jia QB, Fu YY, Cheng NS. Mixed adenoneuroendocrine carcinoma of the gallbladder. Journal of Gastrointestinal Surgery. 2018;**22**(8):1452-1454

[22] La Rosa S, Marando A, Sessa F, Capella C. Mixed adenoneuroendocrine carcinomas (MANECs) of the gastrointestinal tract: An update. Cancers (Basel). 2012;**4**(1):11-30

[23] Ito H, Kudo A, Matsumura S, et al. Mixed adenoneuroendocrine carcinoma of the colon progressed rapidly after hepatic rupture: Report of a case. International Surgery. 2014;**99**(1):40-44

[24] Liu XJ, Feng JS, Xiang WY, et al. Clinicopathological features of an ascending colon mixed adenoneuroendocrine carcinoma with clinical serosal invasion. International Journal of Clinical and Experimental Pathology. 2014;**7**(9):6395-6398

[25] Meşină C, Vasile I, Ciobanu D, et al. Collision tumor of recto-sigmoidian junction – case presentation. Romanian Journal of Morphology and Embryology. 2014;**55**(2 Suppl):643-647

[26] Morais M, Pinho AC, Marques A, et al. Mixed adenoneuroendocrine carcinoma causing colonic intussusception. Case Report Surgery. 2016;**2016**:7684364

[27] Minaya-Bravo AM, Mahillo JCG, et al. Large cell neuroendocrine – adenocarcinoma mixed tumour of colon: Collision tumour with peculiar behaviour. What do we know about these tumours? Annals of Medical Surgery (Lond). 2015;**4**(4):399-403

[28] Shin SH, Kim SH, Jung SH, et al. High-grade mixed adenoneuroendocrine carcinoma in the cecum: A case report. Annals of Coloproctology. 2017;**33**(1):39-42

[29] Peng L, Schwarz RE. Collision tumor in form of primary adenocarcinoma and neuroendocrine carcinoma of the duodenum. Rare Tumors. 2012;**4**(2):e20

[30] Komatsubara T, Koinuma K, Miyakura Y, Horie H, Morimoto M, Ito H, et al. Endocrine cell carcinomas of the colon and rectum: A clinicopathological

evaluation. Clinical Journal of Gastroenterology. 2016;**9**:1-6

[31] Hervieu V, Scoazec JY. Mixed endocrine tumors. Annales de Pathologie. 2005;**25**:511-528

[32] Vanacker L, Smeets D, Hoorens A, Teugels E, Algaba R, Dehou MF, et al. Mixed adenoneuroendocrine carcinoma of the colon: Molecular pathogenesis and treatment. Anticancer Research. 2014;**34**:5517-5521

[33] Tanaka T, Kaneko M, Nozawa H, et al. Diagnosis, assessment, and therapeutic strategy for colorectal mixed adenoneuroendocrine carcinoma. Neuroendocrinology. 2017;**105**(4):426-434

[34] Shah MH, Goldner WS, Benson et al. Neuroendocrine and Adrenal Tumors, Version 2.2021, NCCN Clinical Practice Guidelines in Oncology. Journal of the National Comprehensive Cancer Network. 28 Jul 2021;**19**(7):839-868

Chapter 8

Traumatic Brain Injury: A Review on Some Important Clinical Notes

Behzad Saberi

Abstract

Traumatic brain injury results from any impact on the head, which could disrupt the normal function of the brain. The aim of this review is to evaluate traumatic brain injury from a clinical perspective by pointing to some important clinical notes about traumatic brain injury. The main target groups that this study is designed for are the clinicians who are dealing with patients suffering from traumatic brain injury and also scholars who would like to review some important notes about traumatic brain injury and may want to increase their knowledge about that. This review is designed in a way that would be as concise and informative as possible. This would be of help to review some important notes about the topic in a short period of time.

Keywords: brain, injury, trauma, clinical notes, review

1. Introduction

Traumatic Brain Injury is a common cause of referring patients to the emergency wards and the intensive care units. Head injuries leading to cause damage to the brain tissue and surrounding structures are among the main causes of morbidity and mortality in the communities. Using motor vehicles and machines increases the risk of the occurrence of trauma. This includes causing trauma to the brain and surrounding structures either.

The trauma-related deaths are common in early middle age and youth, and traumatic brain injury contributes in a significant way to the outcome of affected patients. Traumatic brain injury has a wide spectrum, from mild concussions to severe forms of brain injury.

Traumatic brain injuries may be classified into two main groups: the primary and the secondary ones. Treatment strategies may be taken based on this classification. However, new pathophysiology-related studies and relevant findings suggest that in case of necessity, the treatment should be started as soon as possible regardless of considering such classification. In fact, as long as the initial treatment starts earlier, the outcome would become better unless the initial condition of the affected patients is bad enough, which even early initializing the treatment, would not affect the patient's outcome. This is mostly pronounced in the cases of severe traumatic brain injuries and in the persistence of the possible concomitant pathologies that may cause organ failure and death. The same would be pronounced in polytraumatized patients.

The pathologies that may cause traumatic brain injuries include direct trauma to the brain tissue and surrounding structures, brain swelling or cerebral edema, intracerebral shearing, cerebral contusion, intracerebral hemorrhage and hydrocephalus development.

Traumatic brain injuries comprise a wide range of topics. This review tries to point to some of the relevant topics and important notes about traumatic brain injuries.

2. Body

2.1 Some notes about the initial approach to the patients suffering from traumatic brain injuries

The occurrence of traumatic brain injury has different causes like motor vehicle accidents, falls, blunt trauma, etc.

There are various factors that should be considered in the evaluation of patients suffering from traumatic brain injury. Depending on the general condition of the patient and by considering the fact that in which grade the patient would be categorized including mild, moderate or severe, the neurological examination should be done for all of the patients.

In the patients who are categorized in moderate to severe form of injury and ones whose general conditions are unstable and require immediate intervention, first of all, resuscitative efforts should be done including evaluation of the airway, breathing, circulation, disability, exposure and necessary interventions should be done accordingly. After stabilizing the general condition of the patients, evaluation of the traumatic brain injuries should be done.

Neuroimaging including simple Radiography, computed tomography scanning and magnetic resonance imaging is of importance in the initial examination of stabilized patients. Emergency laboratory tests should also be done for all of the admitted patients. In polytraumatized patients, depending on the general condition of the patient, a quick general assessment should be done in search of finding other traumas and fractures, the possible sources of bleeding and obscure blood loss in the patients with hemodynamic instability. In case of possibility, a brief history about the presence of other concomitant disorders in the affected patients should also be done.

In the traumatic brain injury settings, the patients with higher Glasgow coma scale (GCS) generally have better outcomes. A worse outcome may be predicted if the systolic blood pressure is lower than 90 millimeters of mercury or the partial pressure of oxygen is lower than 60 millimeters of mercury. Maintaining the cerebral perfusion pressure in ranges that are higher than 70 millimeters of mercury and trying to keep the intracranial pressure lower than 20 millimeters of mercury should be considered in the affected patients. Controlling the intracranial pressure is an important factor in the management of the patients suffering from traumatic brain injuries. This goal can be achieved by employing various strategies like using paralytics and sedatives, draining the cerebrospinal fluid, coma induction with pentobarbital and administering the mannitol. Administration of mannitol can be done by giving 1 gram per kilogram as a bolus dose and continuing the administration with a route of 0.25 gram per kilogram every 6 hours. In patients suffering from renal failure or congestive heart failure, mannitol should not be administered.

The serum level of the potassium should be kept in the normal range and the patient should be in the normovolemic condition. The occurrence of acute tubular necrosis may be possible during administration of the mannitol, and enough care should be taken to avoid its occurrence by regular checking of the osmolarity of the patient's serum, preferably every 6 hours. In case the osmolarity of the serum falls under 320, administration of the mannitol should be discontinued and be held. Coma induction may be of help to decrease the amount of free radicals, the amount of the cerebral metabolic rate of oxygen and the intracranial pressure. Also, such induction causes myocardial depression, sympathetic tone reduction and hypotension.

Prophylactic measures should be taken against the occurrence of deep vein thrombosis, and the patient's possible high temperature should be controlled. In the epidural hematoma settings, in case the total volume would be lower than 30 cubic centimeters and the thickness would be lower than 15 millimeters with the midline shift, which would be lower than 5 millimeters and in the condition which the patient has a high measured GCS score, the patient can be observed. In such circumstances, neuroimaging should be repeated and the neurological condition of the patient should be examined on a regular basis. Any changes in the patient's condition and new findings in the neuroimaging studies suggesting that the patient's condition is becoming worse should be considered as an emergency, and the neurosurgical intervention should be done as soon as possible [1–3].

There are some classification systems for traumatic brain injuries. Glasgow coma scale or GCS, Mayo and Marshall, are three classification systems that may be used in the evaluation of patients who are suffering from traumatic brain injuries.

In the Glasgow coma scale system, which is commonly used in emergency settings, the patients with traumatic brain injuries would be classified into three main groups including mild, moderate and severe ones.

In the Mayo classification system, traumatic brain injury may be classified into three main groups including possible, mild and moderate to severe ones.

In the Marshall classification system, traumatic brain injury may be classified into six main categories [4–6].

Having knowledge about these three classification systems for evaluation of the patients with traumatic brain injuries can be of help to approach the affected patients with more precision, and this would result in taking an appropriate treatment strategy for the patients based on their conditions and the severity of the traumatic brain injuries.

2.2 Some notes about the respiratory functions and the mechanical ventilation in the patients suffering from traumatic brain injuries

Management of ventilation and oxygenation in traumatic brain injury settings is an important note to be considered at the bedside. Trying to manage the conditions of ventilation and oxygenation in patients suffering from traumatic brain injuries in the first stages is important to reduce the risks for the occurrence of secondary injuries. Also, this management would help improve patient outcomes.

Increased intracranial pressure in patients with traumatic brain injuries is an important problem that these patients encounter. The occurrence of hypocapnia because of the hyperventilation and vasoconstriction in the blood vessels of the brain causes a reduction in the blood flow. As a result, the risk of the occurrence of secondary injuries because of ischemia and hypoperfusion will be increased. In these settings, the recommendation would be to keep the levels of the partial pressure of carbon dioxide in a range between 35 and 40.

Minimizing the bag ventilation of the intubated patients suffering from traumatic brain injuries is an important note which should be kept in mind in reduction of the risk of hyperventilation in these patients. The mechanical ventilator should be employed as early as possible in these patients. Seven to 8 liters per minute may be a reliable starting minute ventilation in these settings. It is because of this fact that there would be a possibility of the existence of the hypermetabolic state in patients suffering from traumatic brain injuries. Since these patients are at risk for developing acute respiratory distress syndrome, permissive hypercapnia is not an appropriate strategy to be taken in these settings.

In such settings, arterial blood gas and capnography should be considered to correlate the end-tidal carbon dioxide with the partial pressure of carbon dioxide. In such circumstances, normoxia is another important parameter. It prevents the occurrence of secondary injury and improves the outcome of the affected patients. About 15–20 minutes after intubation, the arterial blood gas should be checked.

In different cases and based on the curve of the oxygen-hemoglobin dissociation, the ranges for the partial pressure of oxygen in the arterial blood, the fraction of inspired oxygen and the oxygen saturation should be defined.

In patients suffering from traumatic brain injuries, the hemodynamics should be managed appropriately. Any abnormal changes in the blood pressure of these patients should be corrected to prevent further complications [7–9].

The clinicians who are dealing with patients suffering from traumatic brain injuries should have enough knowledge about ventilation and oxygenation management as an important factor in determining the outcome of the patients.

One of the important factors in the management of the patients with traumatic brain injuries, specifically the severe forms of such injuries, would be employing mechanical ventilation. Having enough knowledge to work with the ventilator and relevant terms and physiology is important in traumatic brain injury settings. It is recommended that clinicians who are dealing with patients suffering from traumatic brain injuries, specifically ones who are required to be put on the ventilator, to gain enough knowledge about the lung physiology and details to work with the ventilator [10–12].

2.3 Evaluation of the polytraumatized patients including the traumatic brain injuries with the trauma score

Paying attention to a score called trauma score is of importance in patients suffering from traumatic brain injuries, since the affected patients may have traumas in different parts of the body. So, considering the trauma score would be of help in evaluating the affected patients in a more comprehensive way. Polytraumatized patients with traumatic brain injuries may be evaluated with the trauma score more comprehensively. Having knowledge about the trauma score is of importance to assess polytraumatized patients including those with traumatic brain injuries [13–15].

2.4 Some notes about the skull base fractures in traumatic brain injuries

The patients suffering from traumatic brain injuries may have skull base fractures, which such fractures are of importance and require taking certain strategies in the management of the patients.

Temporal bone skull base fractures are among this category of fractures. Facial palsy, otorrhea, tinnitus, vertigo, postauricular hemorrhage and hemotympanum are the signs of the middle cranial skull base fractures. To classify the temporal bone fractures, the long axis of the petrous pyramid would be used.

The skull base fractures that traverse the middle ear or the paranasal sinuses can be associated with the occurrence of tearing in the dura and may be accompanied by a cerebrospinal fluid fistula. The occurrence of the cerebrospinal fluid fistula can be seen in about 10–20 percent of the patients with skull base fractures. In young children the formation of the cerebrospinal fluid fistula is not common because of the late maturation and development of the paranasal sinuses.

In comparison with the middle and posterior cranial fossae, the anterior fossa where cerebrospinal fluid leaks commonly happen. In the skull base trauma settings there are some indications for surgical repair of the cerebrospinal fluid fistula.

In spite of lumbar drainage, in case the cerebrospinal fluid leakage lasts for more than 7–10 days after the occurrence of the injury, conservative therapy would not be effective and surgical repair should be done for the cerebrospinal fluid leakage.

Having a high risk for meningitis development, the presence of the pneumocephalus and the large dural tear, delayed cerebrospinal fluid leakage, penetrating injuries and external brain herniation are the indications for early surgical intervention.

The swelling of the frontal lobe will be decreased in a time period of about 10 days after the occurrence of the trauma. It allows enough retraction to expose the anterior skull base. Traumatic otorrhea will be resolved in about 14 days after the time of the injury, and therefore, surgical repair is usually not necessary in such circumstances. Therefore, the conservative management of the cerebrospinal fluid otorrhea should be considered for longer periods after the injury. Just in case conservative management fails, the surgical intervention can be considered.

In the traumatic brain injury settings, skull base injuries are important and should be focused on in the treatment of patients suffering from traumatic brain injuries [16–21].

3. Conclusion

Traumatic brain injury, as a neurological insult due to trauma, is a common cause of referring patients to the emergency wards and the intensive care units. It is important for clinicians, specifically neurosurgeons, neurologists, intensivists and emergency medicine physicians to have enough knowledge about various aspects of traumatic brain injuries. Having such knowledge is important to approach the affected patients with more precision at the bedside.

In the management of patients with traumatic brain injuries, paying enough attention to details is crucial. Traumatic brain injury comprises a wide range of topics, and any of them includes important notes.

Considering these, it is recommended to study more about the traumatic brain injuries and relevant topics from other sources until getting familiar with various aspects of traumatic brain injuries and the relevant important notes.

Conflict of interest

The author declares no conflict of interest.

Author details

Behzad Saberi
Independent Medical Researcher, Esfahan, Iran

*Address all correspondence to: sab64b@yahoo.com

References

[1] Dixon J, Comstock G, Whitfield J, Richards D, Burkholder TW, Leifer N, et al. Emergency department management of traumatic brain injuries: A resource tiered review. African Journal of Emergency Medicine. 2020;**10**(3):159-166

[2] Capizzi A, Woo J, Verduzco-Gutierrez M. Traumatic brain injury. Medical Clinics of North America. 2020;**104**(2):213-238

[3] Robinson CP. Moderate and severe traumatic brain injury. Continuum: Lifelong Learning in Neurology. 2021;**27**(5):1278-1300

[4] Helmy A, Vizcaychipi M, Gupta A. Traumatic brain injury: Intensive care management. British Journal of Anaesthesia. 2007;**99**(1):32-42

[5] Malec JF, Brown AW, Leibson CL, Flaada JT, Mandrekar JN, Diehl NN, et al. The Mayo classification system for traumatic brain injury severity. Journal of Neurotrauma. 2007;**24**(9):1417-1424

[6] Marshall LF, Marshall SB, Klauber MR, Clark MVB, Eisenberg HM, Jane JA, et al. A new classification of head injury based on computerized tomography. Journal of Neurosurgery. 1991;**75**(Supplement):S14-S20

[7] Carney N, Totten AM, O'Reilly C, Ullman JS, Hawryluk GW, Bell MJ, et al. Guidelines for the management of severe traumatic brain injury, fourth edition. Neurosurgery. 2017;**80**(1):6-15

[8] Pelosi P, Ferguson ND, Frutos-Vivar F, Anzueto A, Putensen C, Raymondos K, et al. Management and outcome of mechanically ventilated neurologic patients*. Critical Care Medicine. 2011;**39**(6):1482-1492

[9] Davis DP, Idris AH, Sise MJ, Kennedy F, Eastman AB, Velky T, et al. Early ventilation and outcome in patients with moderate to severe traumatic brain injury*. Critical Care Medicine. 2006;**34**(4):1202-1208

[10] Pham T, Brochard LJ, Slutsky AS. Mechanical ventilation: State of the art. Mayo Clinic Proceedings. 2017;**92**(9):1382-1400

[11] Weingart SD. Managing initial mechanical ventilation in the emergency department. Annals of Emergency Medicine. 2016;**68**(5):614-617

[12] Singer BD, Corbridge TC. Basic invasive mechanical ventilation. Southern Medical Journal. 2009;**102**(12):1238-1245

[13] Gilpin D, Nelson P. Revised trauma score: A triage tool in the accident and emergency department. Injury. 1991;**22**(1):35-37

[14] Long WB, Bachulis BL, Hynes GD. Accuracy and relationship of mechanisms of injury, trauma score, and injury severity score in identifying major trauma. The American Journal of Surgery. 1986;**151**(5):581-584

[15] Champion HR, Sacco WJ, Carnazzo AJ, Copes W, Fouty WJ. Trauma score. Critical Care Medicine. 1981;**9**(9):672-676

[16] Ishman SL, Friedland DR. Temporal bone fractures: Traditional classification and clinical relevance. The Laryngoscope. 2004;**114**(10):1734-1741

[17] Gordts F, Foulon I, Hachimi-Idrissi S. Basilar skull fractures: The petrous bone. B-ENT. 2016;**Suppl. 26**(1):193-201

[18] Baugnon KL, Hudgins PA. Skull base fractures and their complications. Neuroimaging Clinics of North America. 2014;**24**(3):439-465

[19] Zapalac JS, Marple BF, Schwade ND. Skull base cerebrospinal fluid fistulas: A comprehensive diagnostic algorithm. Otolaryngology–Head and Neck Surgery. 2002;**126**(6):669-676

[20] Meco C, Oberascher G. Comprehensive algorithm for skull base dural lesion and cerebrospinal fluid fistula diagnosis. The Laryngoscope. 2004;**114**(6):991-999

[21] Phang SY, Whitehouse K, Lee L, Khalil H, McArdle P, Whitfield PC. Management of CSF leak in base of skull fractures in adults. British Journal of Neurosurgery. 2016;**30**(6):596-604

Section 3

Supportive Treatment Approaches in Global Diseases

Chapter 9

Exploring the Therapeutic Potential from *Moringa oleifera* and *Urtica dioica* Bioactive Compounds in Managing Diabetes and Insulin Resistance

Hanane Moummou, Jamal Karoumi, Mounir Tilaoui, Es-Said Sabir, Imane Meftah, Mounia Achoch, Hicham Chatoui, Omar El Hiba and Lahoucine Bahi

Abstract

Diabetes is one of the ubiquitous metabolic disorders, indicating increasing chronic blood levels (chronic hyperglycaemia). Its three types are mostly caused by different pathogenic conditions (disorders in the secretion and/or regulation blood sugar insulin levels), often resulting from defects in insulin secretion and abnormal glucose tolerance. In addition, most people with diabetes have type 2 diabetes, which is characterised by insulin resistance and progressive beta-cell failure. Recently, there has been a growing demand for medicinal plants traditionally used to manage diabetes and its complications, as the insulin use is somewhat correlated with side effects. The current chapter focused on two medicinal plants, *Moringa oleifera* and *Urtica dioica*. The chosen plants have shown therapeutic potential as natural diabetes remedies owing to their bioactive compounds. The chosen plants have shown potential as natural diabetes remedies owing to their diverse bioactive compounds range and their effect on insulin resistance and glucose levels. Additionally, they exhibit hypoglycaemic features making them promising candidates for further diabetes management investigation. Besides, because of their bioactive phytochemicals, they do have the ability to prevent the diabetes's onset. Of note, this chapter aims to explore their effects on blood sugar regulation with a focus on managing diabetes potential.

Keywords: insulin, insulin resistance, diabetes, blood glucose, bioactive compounds, *Moringa oleifera*, *Urtica dioica*

1. Introduction

Diabetes and insulin resistance are two common health problems affecting large numbers of people around the world and understanding them is essential to managing them effectively.

On the one hand, the World Health Organization reports that around 537 million adults aged 20–79 will be living with diabetes worldwide in 2021. Moreover, insulin resistance is a precursor to type 2 diabetes, which occurs when the body's cells become less reactive to insulin.

Furthermore, to combat this disease, researchers are making enormous efforts, both in the field of medical biotechnology through drugs and in the phytotherapeutic field and natural compounds through medicinal plants, which have proved highly effective in both prevention and treatment.

This chapter aims to elucidate the therapeutic potential of two anti-diabetic plants, *Moringa oleifera* and *Urtica dioica*. *Moringa oleifera* is rich in bioactive compounds, notably antioxidants, phytosterols, and isothiocyanates, while *Urtica dioica* contains phenolic compounds, flavonoids, and triterpenes. These compounds have a hypoglycemic effect, making them valuable for the prevention and treatment of diabetes.

2. Chemical composition of *Moringa oleifera* and Urtica

Aromatic plants (or medicinal herbs) have been used for centuries in traditional medicine [1] and culinary practices due to their potential health benefits. These aromatic plants can be used in various ways, including teas, essential oils, culinary dishes, and herbal remedies [2]. Among these aromatic plants, we find *Moringa oleifera* and *Urtica*, which are known for their medicinal properties [3]. *Urtica* and *Moringa* are two different plants with distinct chemical compositions. Here is an overview of each chemical composition.

2.1 Phytochemicals

The bioactive compounds found in aromatic plants correspond to compounds synthesized by plants and are sometimes present in conjugated forms as glycosides. They originate from the plant's secondary metabolism and act against environmental aggressions [4]. These compounds are divided into five major categories: flavonoids, phenolic acids, lignans, stilbenes, and tannins, most of which are derived from the polymerization of flavonoids. Polyphenols are molecules that have several phenolic groups, meaning they have an aromatic ring with one or more hydroxyl (-OH) groups attached. Both *Moringa oleifera* and *Urtica* contain a variety of bioactive compounds including flavonoids, phenolic compounds, and sterols.

Moringa leaves are indeed an excellent source of vitamins and minerals, including vitamin C, vitamin A, vitamin K, calcium, iron, and potassium [5]. *Urtica* is also a good source of vitamins and minerals, but the content may not be as high as in *Moringa* [6]. Both plants are a source of high-quality plant proteins, containing all essential amino acids, making them useful for supplementing protein intake [7]. Additionally, they are rich in dietary fiber, which can promote good digestive health.

Regarding bioactive compounds, *Moringa oleifera* contains over 100 compounds. It is rich in antioxidants such as flavonoids, polyphenols, and quercetin (**Figure 1**) which help combat damage caused by free radicals in the body. Its chemical composition also shows the presence of phytosterols and plant compounds like cholesterol,

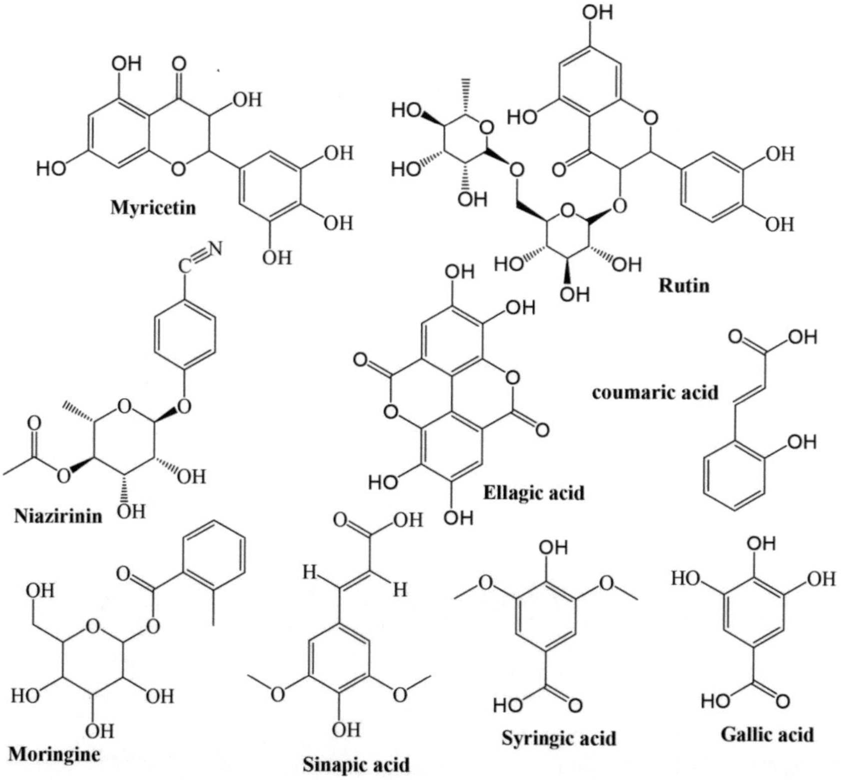

Figure 1.
Some bioactive compounds in Moringa oleifera (MO) [8]. This figure illustrates the diversity of bioactive compounds present in Moringa. These compounds display a variety of structural features, including aromatic rings and bicyclic structures with different substituents. The presence of these compounds underlines Moringa's potential as a functional food, suggesting that it is suitable for a wide range of applications in the promotion of health and well-being.

which can help reduce blood cholesterol levels. Other studies have shown that *Moringa* leaves contain glucosinolates with anticancer properties, as well as isothiocyanates that can be used as anti-inflammatories.

Stinging nettles contain lignans like secoisolariciresinol [9], which have potential health benefits, and tannins, which may have unique health benefits, particularly in traditional herbal medicine [10]. In addition to these compounds, studies show that *Urtica* is rich in phenolic compounds, flavonoids, triterpenes, coumarin, and sterols like beta-sitosterol (**Figure 2**).

Finally, studies on the chemical composition of *Moringa* [8] and *Urtica* [11] show that there are several common compounds (**Figure 3**) between these two plants. These common compounds are found in both plants but with varying concentrations.

2.2 Fatty acids

It is worth adding that the essential oil extracted from *Moringa* and *Urtica* seeds is rich in monounsaturated and polyunsaturated fatty acids [12, 13], such as oleic acid and linoleic acid, which are "beneficial for cardiovascular health."

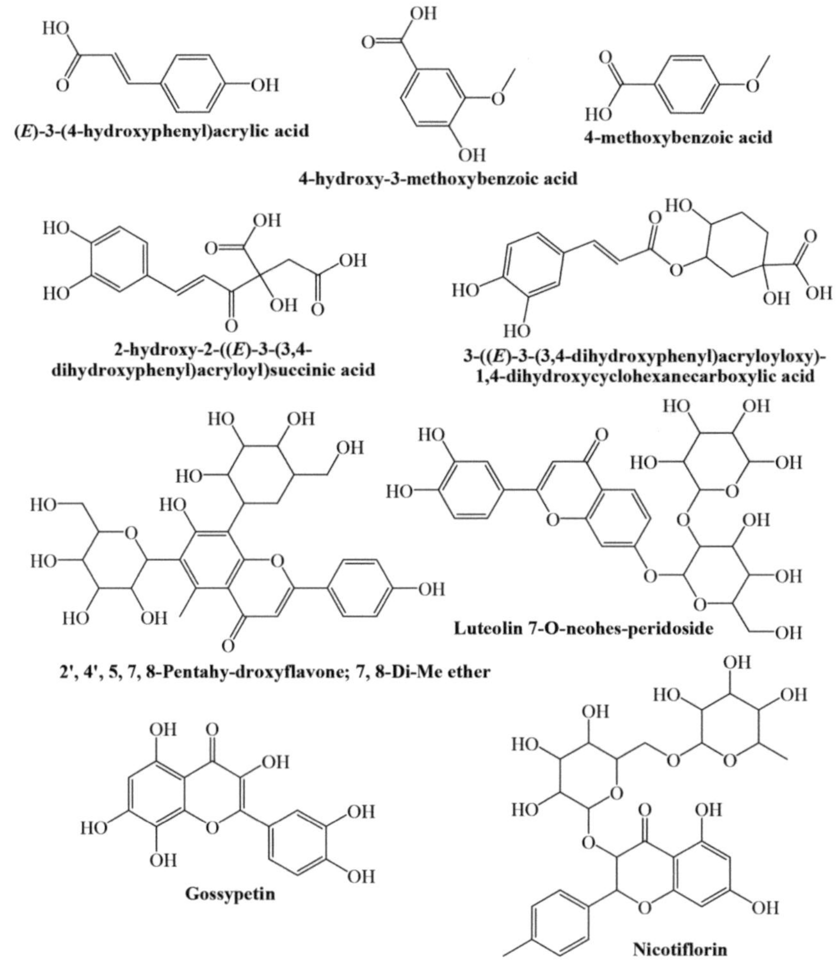

Figure 2.
Some bioactive compounds isolated from Urtica dioica (UD) [11]. The figure highlights the main aromatic compounds present in Urtica, also known as stinging nettle. These compounds encompass a wide range of phytochemicals, the most notable representatives of which are flavonoids and phenolic acids. Flavonoids and phenolic acids are well known for their medicinal properties, notably their antioxidant, anti-inflammatory and antimicrobial effects. These constituents are highly valued in traditional phytotherapy for their therapeutic potential. Urtica is traditionally used for its antiviral activities and anti-inflammatory properties. The antiviral effects are particularly important, as they contribute to Urtica's ability to fight viral infections. In addition, its anti-inflammatory properties help relieve inflammatory conditions such as arthritis and allergies. Overall, the presence of these aromatic compounds in Urtica underlines its medicinal importance and supports its traditional use as a remedy for a variety of ailments.

2.2.1 Diabetes

Diabetes is a multifaceted condition closely linked to disturbances in insulin metabolism. This section aims to elucidate the chronological progression, diagnostic procedures, associated complications, and diabetes therapeutic approaches to promote a more comprehensive understanding of this disease. Moreover, the synthesis of the information presented here is summarized in **Figure 1**, which delineates the different stages of diabetes based on dynamic changes in the functionality of pancreatic β-cells, which play an essential role in the secretion of the hormone insulin. Besides the insulin resistance effect on diabetes complications, other hormones are implied in the blood's unbalanced glucose concentration, especially cortisol and ghrelin.

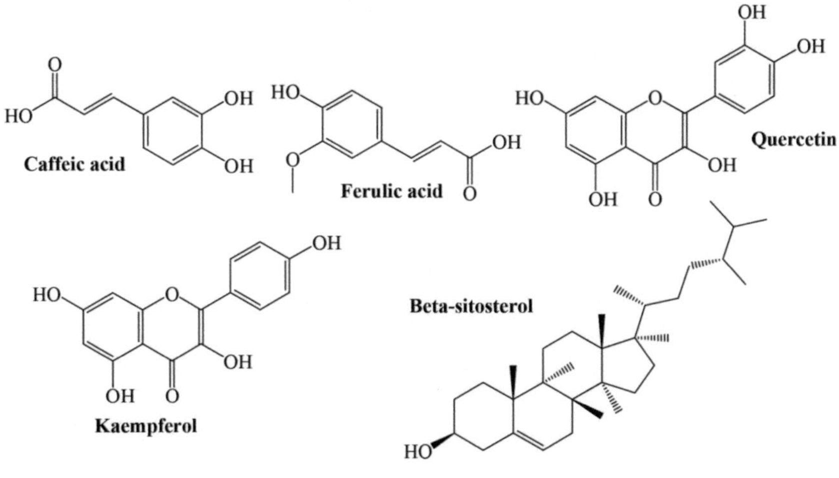

Figure 3.
Some of MO and UD common compounds. These compounds' illustrations give a concise overview of the compounds common to Moringa and Urtica. Phenolic acids and polyphenols are the predominant products in both plants, demonstrating their importance in terms of bioactive constituents. However, it should be noted that these compounds exist in varying concentrations in each plant species. This variation in concentration suggests that while Moringa and Urtica share common compounds, their compositions may differ, which could influence their individual therapeutic properties and applications.

2.2.2 Diabetes pathogenesis

According to the World Health Organization (WHO), in 1999, diabetes mellitus was defined as "multiple aetiology's metabolic disorder which is caused by chronic hyperglycaemia accompanied by disorders of carbohydrate, lipid and protein metabolism resulting from abnormalities in insulin secretion, insulin action or both of them," Nevertheless, insulin, a hormone produced by the islet cells of the pancreas, and glucagon, another hormone produced by the α cells of the pancreas, together regulate blood sugar levels [14]. Besides, high blood sugar levels trigger the release of insulin, which activates carbohydrates' absorption, particularly glucose, via specific receptors in the muscles, adipose tissue, and liver. Additionally, two main pathogenic pathways contribute to chronic hyperglycaemia in diabetes: (i) destruction of β-cells leading to insufficient insulin production, and (ii) insufficient insulin action due to deficient insulin secretion and/or defects in insulin reactivity. Moreover, prolonged elevation of blood glucose levels can cause damage to various organs, including the eyes, kidneys, nerves, heart, and blood vessels.

2.2.3 Diabetes's types

The World Health Organization (WHO) has first delineated diabetes into the following clinical categories [15]:

2.2.3.1 Type 1 diabetes

The first one or type 1 diabetes, results from the destruction of β-cells, usually leading to absolute insulin deficiency. The latter is an immune-mediated process (referred to as type 1A). Although a small subset of cases present with an idiopathic form of the disease (identified as type 1B). Its main clinical features include a sudden onset at a young age (before 35), a normal body mass index (BMI), the introduction of insulin within 12 months of diagnosis, and an increased risk of diabetic ketoacidosis [16]. This form accounts for 5–10% of cases of diabetes.

2.2.3.2 Type 2 diabetes

Til 95% of diabetes cases belong to type 2, which arises owing to cell dysfunction, leading to a progressive insulin secretion loss amidst insulin resistance [15]. This diabetes's category onset is gradual and typically occurs at a later age which is notably distinct point from type 1. In addition, most individuals with this kind of diabetes are overweight or obese. Besides, they are less likely to require insulin treatment within 12 months of diagnosis, and they do not present ketoacidosis [16].

2.2.3.3 Gestational diabetes mellitus (GDM)

GDM is diagnosed during pregnancy, especially in the second or third trimester. Typically, it disappears after delivery, but some type 2 diabetes cases may be identified during pregnancy [15]. Overweight status, older age, family history of diabetes, or a personal history of GDM are the main risk factors. Nevertheless, lifestyle interventions and insulin injections may mitigate adverse pregnancy outcomes such as macrocosmic infants and preeclampsia.

2.2.3.4 Specific diabetes type (SDT)

This diabetes class may arise from a tremendous condition not encompassed within the previous ones. Nevertheless, included in this category are as follows:

- ailments affecting the exocrine pancreas,
- endocrine disorders,
- chemically induced diabetes (resulting from the administration of glucocorticoids or antifungals, e.g., pentamidine),
- infections,
- single-gene abnormalities impacting β-cell function,
- monogenic defects in insulin action,
- various genetic syndromes associated with diabetes such as Down syndrome or Klinefelter syndrome [16].

2.2.3.5 Diabetes's hybrid forms

This last one was considered by the World Health Organization (WHO) as a "Hybrid Forms of Diabetes," which incorporates clinical presentations that amalgamate characteristics from both type 1 and type 2 diabetes [15]. Besides, it accommodates conditions such as slowly progressive immune-mediated diabetes, previously referred to as latent autoimmune diabetes in adults (LADA), where clinical features mirror those of type 2

DOI: http://dx.doi.org/10.5772/intechopen.1004618

diabetes, yet individuals display pancreatic autoantibodies. Additionally, ketosis-prone type 2 diabetes might be considered as "example for this diabetes type."

2.2.4 Diagnostic profile

Globally, the diabetes's classic symptoms include polyuria, polydipsia, fatigue, and weakness. In type 1 diabetes, these symptoms may also be accompanied by weight loss despite an increased appetite and occasional blurred vision. Notably, type 1 diabetes symptoms tend to manifest rapidly within days or weeks, making it less likely that they will be detected during routine medical screenings [16].

Conversely, the onset of diabetes's type 2 onset often transpires without overt clinical manifestations, necessitating diagnoses during routine examinations. Beyond the conventional symptoms of diabetes, type 2 cases may manifest additional conditions such as skin infections or impaired wound healing. An estimated one-third of patients diagnosed with type 2 diabetes already present chronic complications at the diagnosis point.

2.2.4.1 Blood test for diabetes diagnosis (DD)

According to the diabetes diagnosis of WHO [17], the distinct advantages and insights related to the four prevalent blood tests employed for diagnosing diabetes and prediabetes are illustrated in **Table 1**.

2.2.5 Treatment

2.2.5.1 Lifestyle management

Firstly, embracing a health-conscious lifestyle serves as a cornerstone for both preventing diabetes and mitigating its potential complications [16]. Secondly, every meal should contain a carbohydrate, while adhering to principles of moderation regarding fat intake.

Nevertheless, by incorporating complex carbohydrates strategically across meals while factoring in the glycaemic index, diabetic individuals can ensure sustained energy levels while minimizing blood sugar spikes [21].

Owing to the increasing role of physical activity, the World Health Organization (WHO) generally recommends 150 minutes of moderate-intensity physical activity or 75 minutes per week of vigorous activity, which is recommended per week, tailored to the individual's age and capabilities. It might also help control blood sugar, reduce cardiovascular risk factors, and enhance overall well-being and mental health [20].

Because cardiovascular disease, premature mortality, and microvascular complications are major risk factors for smokers, individuals with diabetes are strongly encouraged to abstain from tobacco use [21].

2.2.5.2 Pharmacological treatment

2.2.5.2.1 Pharmacological type 1 diabetes treatment

Besides, the last one might result from combinations of intermediate or long action with rapid action. Moreover, people with type 1 diabetes need insulin treatment to survive (**Table 2**) [22].

Blood test	Features	Conditions and %
Hemoglobin A1c (HbA1c)	• Simply performed. • Diabetes and prediabetes diagnosis. • Linked to the glucose percentage which is attached to hemoglobin.	• No prior fasting required. • Blood sugar indicator. • Not affected by stress [18]. • 6.5 and between 5.7 and 6.4 are, respectively, related to diabetes and prediabetes [19].
The plasma glucose (PG) value at any time	• Similar diabetes symptoms	• No prior fasting required • 11.1 mmol/l (200 mg/dl)
The oral glucose tolerance test (OGTT)	• DD • PG measurement	• 2 hours after taking syrup containing 75 grams of glucose. • 7.8 and 11 mmol/l (140–199 mg/dl) for PG = [glucose intolerance] [19].
The fasting glucose test (FAG)	• DD	• Measuring venous PG levels after 8 hours fasting. • DD measurements (twice) test is 7 mmol/l (≥126 mg/dl). • 6.1 and 6.9 mmol/l (110–125 mg/dl) according to WHO. • 5.6 and 6.9 mmol/l (100–125 mg/dl) according to American Diabetes Association (ADA) [20].

***Table** 1 explains that hemoglobin A1c (HbA1c) is a simple test used to diagnose diabetes and prediabetes. It measures the percentage of glucose bound to hemoglobin in the blood over time. Unlike other tests, it does not require fasting. HbA1c serves as an indicator of blood glucose levels and is not affected by stress. A result of 6.5 or more indicates diabetes, while a result between 5.7 and 6.4 indicates pre-diabetes. Besides, the plasma glucose (PG) value at any given time is a measure of glucose concentration in the blood. It presents symptoms like those of diabetes and does not require fasting before testing. A plasma glucose level of 11.1 mmol/l (200 mg/dl) or more indicates diabetes. The oral glucose tolerance test (OGTT) is a diagnostic test for diabetes. It involves measuring plasma glucose levels 2 hours after consuming a syrup containing 75 grams of glucose. If plasma glucose levels are between 7.8 and 11 mmol/l (140–199 mg/dl), this indicates glucose intolerance, which is a precursor to diabetes. The fasting plasma glucose test is a diagnostic test for diabetes. It involves measuring the glucose level in venous plasma after an 8-hour fasting period. A diagnosis of diabetes is made if the plasma glucose level is equal to or greater than 7 mmol/l (≥126 mg/dl) on two separate occasions. According to the World Health Organization (WHO), a fasting blood glucose level between 6.1 and 6.9 mmol/l (110–125 mg/dl) indicates impaired fasting glucose, while the American Diabetes Association (ADA) defines this range as between 5.6 and 6.9 mmol/l (100–125 mg/dl) [20].*

Table 1.
Blood glucose tests features.

2.2.5.2.2 Pharmacological type 2 diabetes treatment

Managing diabetes type 2 primarily involves both dietary and lifestyle modifications.

Pharmacological intervention becomes necessary when glycaemic targets remain unattained, typically commencing with metformin, an oral hypoglycaemic agent belonging to the biguanide class [20]. According to French recommendations outlined

Insulin type	Features	Conditions
Fast-acting insulin	Action begins approximately 15 minutes after injection	Peaking at 1 hour and having effects for 2–4 hours
Intermediate-acting insulin	Its action begins between 2 and 4 hours after injection	Its peak is reached in 4–12 hours, and it is effective for 12–18 hours
Long-acting insulin	It reaches the bloodstream within a few hours of injection	Its action lasts 24 hours or more, without peak

***Table** 2 explains that the fast-acting insulin starts to work around 15 minutes after injection, with a peak at 1 hour and effects for 2–4 hours. Intermediate-acting insulin begins to act between 2 and 4 hours after injection, with a peak reached between 4 and 12 hours, and remains effective for 12–18 hours. Long-acting insulin reaches the bloodstream a few hours after injection, and its action lasts 24 hours or more, with no pronounced peak.*

Table 2.
Insulin's categories.

by the High Authority of Health (HAS), this initial stage is defined as "monotherapy" [23]. In contrast, when glycaemic goals are not met, practitioners must introduce another medication, which allows "dual therapy by metformin and sulfonylurea combination."

A third hypoglycaemic agent medication, either oral (such as alpha-glucosidase inhibitors, gliptins, or gliflozin's) or injectable (either insulin or glucagon-like peptide-1 [GLP-1] analogs) could be added when blood sugar levels could not decrease. Besides, patients with advanced stage, may combine "intermediate- or long-acting insulin" along with rapid-acting insulin.

Besides, controlling glucose levels remains essential for the human body balance owing to the pancreas's beta cells generating the hypoglycaemic hormone. Besides, this glucose metabolism steadiness could be reestablished by exploring its homeostasis regulation ways and consequences upon the pathological paths [24].

3. Insulin resistance and diabetes

Insulin resistance is a key pathophysiological and a powerful predictor of future type 2 diabetes mellitus, and metabolic syndrome is the foremost therapeutic target in the treatment of hyperglycaemia (**Figure 4**) [25]. Current research has shown that natural products including *Moringa oleifera* (commonly known as drumstick tree) and *Urtica dioica* (commonly known as stinging nettle) have promising beneficial effects on insulin resistance.

3.1 *Moringa oleifera's* impacts upon insulin resistance and diabetes

3.1.1 Moringa oleifera's effect upon insulin resistance

Moringa oleifera has gained a lot of attention in recent years due to its potential health benefits in managing insulin resistance, a condition associated with metabolic disorders and type 2 diabetes [26]. Various scientific research and studies have investigated the impact of *Moringa oleifera* on insulin resistance and have shown promising results.

Amelia et al. carried out the impact of *Moringa oleifera* on insulin levels and folliculogenesis in a polycystic ovary syndrome model rats with insulin resistance.

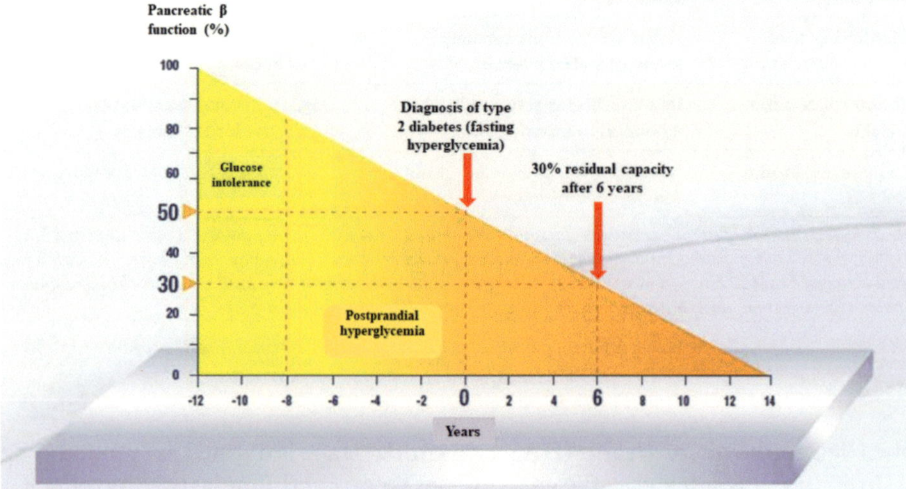

Figure 4.
Correlation between β-cell function and diabetes evolution: insulin resistance and impaired insulin secretion are two key factors in the development of type 2 diabetes (T2D). These factors often manifest themselves in people with pre-diabetes and progressively worsen over time. At the time of diagnosis, pancreatic beta-cell function is generally around 50% of normal, with an annual decline of around 5%. Research suggests that the decline in beta-cell function begins around 10–12 years before diagnosis, and by 6 years after diagnosis, it can fall to less than 25% of normal function. This highlights the progressive nature of β-cell dysfunction in the development and progression of T2DM.

The results showed that rats fed with *Moringa oleifera* extract showed an improvement in insulin sensitivity through increasing insulin signaling, leading to better glucose uptake and regulating folliculogenesis, thus managing insulin resistance associated with polycystic ovary syndrome [27]. Similarly, Divi et al. [28] investigate the potential therapeutic effects on diabetes and hyperlipidemia in insulin resistance rats. The study compares the effects of *Moringa oleifera* extract in streptozotocin-induced diabetes rats and insulin resistance in rats fed with a high-fructose diet. The results demonstrate that the aqueous extract of *Moringa oleifera* improves insulin sensitivity and regulates glucose levels, which could be crucial for treating polycystic ovary syndrome. Also, it ameliorates serum lipid profiles and corrects abdominal fat content [28]. Additionally, Siahaan et al. explore the effect of *Moringa oleifera* leaves on insulin and glucose levels in *Rattus norvegicus* polycystic ovary syndrome model. The study shows an enhancement in insulin levels, insulin sensitivity improvement, and regulation of glucose homeostasis in *Moringa oleifera* leaves treated rats (**Table 3**) [31].

Moreover, accumulating studies explore the impact of isothiocyanate-rich extract from *Moringa oleifera* extract on hepatic glucogenesis, weight gain, and insulin resistance in mice. Those results show that isothiocyanate-rich extract from *Moringa oleifera* inhibits hepatic glucogenesis, which is important in managing blood glucose levels, especially for those with insulin resistance. Furthermore, the extract has a significant effect on alleviating insulin resistance in HepG2 cells via enhancing glucose uptake modulation insulin signaling pathways and improving insulin sensitivity and glucose metabolism through activation of the AMPK pathway, a key player in regulating cellular energy balance [30, 32, 33]. Similarly, Gu et al. found that crud polysaccharides from *Moringa oleifera* improve insulin resistance in HepG2

Parameter	*Moringa oleifera*	*Urtica dioica*
Insulin sensitivity (IS)	Improves IS through increasing glucose uptake and insulin signaling pathways	Enhances IS via several molecular mechanisms, such as inhibition of inflammatory pathways and decreasing adiposity
Glucose homeostasis	Control blood glucose levels (BGL) through utilization and stimulation glucose uptake	Participate in the regulation of BGL by reducing insulin resistance-related metabolic and improving pancreatic β-cell function
Oxidative stress (OS)	Mitigates OS associated with insulin resistance	Decreasing OS, preserve and restore β-cell function
Inflammation (IM)	Decreases systemic IM and inhibits inflammatory pathways associated to insulin resistance	Improves insulin sensitivity by suppressing IM processes linked to insulin resistance.
Adiposity (AD)	Impairment of insulin resistance through AD reduction	Improves insulin sensitivity via decreasing AD and adipose tissue inflammation
Pancreatic function	Enhances pancreatic β-cell function and insulin production	Ameliorates insulin secretion, enhances glucose homeostasis, and improves β-cell function and glucose tolerance
Lipid metabolism (LM)	Reduces dyslipidemia, improves LM and regulates lipid metabolism profiles	Improves metabolism, decrease lipid levels and exhibits hypolipidemic activities

From this table, it demonstrates that Moringa oleifera and Urtica dioica both have beneficial effects on diabetes-related parameters. Moringa oleifera improves insulin sensitivity by enhancing glucose uptake and insulin signaling pathways, while Urtica dioica improves insulin sensitivity by inhibiting inflammatory pathways and reducing adiposity. Both plants contribute to glucose homeostasis, with Moringa oleifera promoting glucose utilization and absorption and Urtica dioica regulating blood sugar levels by reducing problems associated with insulin resistance and improving pancreatic β-cell function. In addition, they both alleviate the oxidative stress associated with insulin resistance, reduce inflammation, improve pancreatic function, and regulate lipid metabolism. Moringa oleifera reduces dyslipidaemia and improves lipid metabolism profiles, while Urtica dioica decreases lipid levels and exhibits hypolipidemic activities.

Table 3.
Effect of Moringa oleifera and Urtica dioica on insulin resistance [29, 30].

cells [34]. Additionally, another study conducted by Afifah et al. demonstrates that *Moringa oleifera* extract alleviates insulin resistance through increasing insulin and GLUT-2 expression in pancreatic islet cells, showing its potential therapeutic effects on improving insulin sensitivity and enhancing pancreatic β-cell function, ensuring an appropriate amount of insulin production, and improving pancreatic glucose sensing [35]. Moreover, molecular docking studies revealed that *Moringa oleifera* compounds interacted effectively with insulin tyrosine kinase receptors, showing its potential therapeutic effects on modulating insulin signaling pathways and managing diabetes [36].

3.1.2 Moringa oleifera's effect upon diabetes

Of note, both phenolic and flavonoid *Moringa*'s compounds tested aqueous extract (MTAE) regenerate the pancreas's β-cells, which boosts insulin secretion [37]. In the second one's case, their oxidative activity's inhibition is due to proton donors. Also, carotenoids and phenolic compounds are among *Moringa's* leaves' phytochemicals. Besides, lipid peroxidation is prevented by antioxidants *Moringa* plant peroxyl radicals, while the ability to trap elements such as hydroxyl radicals is attributed to phenolic compounds [38]. Considering glucose, whether in hypoglycemia or hyperglycemia, with insulin levels which are inversely proportional, on the first hand, they are a condition where the blood glucose levels are respectively less than 60 mg/dl and more than 180 mg/dl. On the other hand, organs might be damaged when their concentration is higher than 125 mg/dl. For this, extra insulin doses decrease blood sugar levels and prevent the consequent glucose level complications fluctuations. Back to phototherapeutics implication, being considered as the best medicinal plant, *Moringa oleifera* could help combat a tremendous disease, especially diabetes mellitus [39]. Furthermore, thanks to their phytochemicals, *Moringa* leaves significantly affect pancreatic insulin. Among them, antioxidants can prevent lipid peroxidation, as mentioned above. These nutraceuticals are involved in preventing diabetes mellitus onset, progression, and complications [39].

3.2 *Urtica dioica's* impacts upon insulin resistance and diabetes

3.2.1 Urtica dioica and insulin resistance

Urtica dioica, commonly known as stinging nettle, has been studied for its potential health benefits, such as insulin resistance, suggesting the potential effect of this plant in improving glucose metabolism and preventing type 2 diabetes [40, 41]. *Urtica dioica* contains a variety of bioactive compounds, including lectins, phenolic acids, triterpenes, sterols, and flavonoids, which have shown antioxidant, anti-inflammatory, and antidiabetic activities [42]. Various studies have explored the effects of *Urtica dioica* on diabetes and insulin resistance. Shahrokhi through a randomized controlled trial, showed a significant reduction in HbA1c levels in the *Urtica dioica* treated group compared to the placebo group. This study suggests that *Urtica dioica* could be used as adjunctive therapy in type 1 diabetes mellitus as it demonstrates a positive impact on preserving pancreatic β-cell function and enhancing insulin sensitivity via the reduction in HbA1c [43]. Fan also investigates the potential use of *Urtica dioica* in mitigating insulin resistance and fat accumulation using a prediabetic mouse model. The result showed an increase in insulin sensitivity and an improvement in glucose tolerance in mice fed with *Urtica dioica*, indicating its promising role in managing metabolic syndrome such as diabetes [29]. In addition, *Urtica dioica* extract exhibits a significant amelioration in insulin sensitivity in obese mice through inhibition of PP2A activity, which phosphorylates insulin receptor substrates, leading to enhanced glucose uptake and insulin signaling pathways in skeletal muscle cells [44]. Another study found that *Urtica dioica* leaf extract stimulates insulin secretion in isolated islets of Langerhans cells an improves glucose tolerance in streptozotocin-induced diabetic rats, suggesting its potential therapeutic role in treating diabetes [45].

3.2.2 Urtica dioica and diabetes

Nettle has several properties related to insulin, such as insulin sensitivity and secretagogue. It also has several properties related to insulin such as being insulin-sensitiviting and secretagogue. In addition, the intestine is the starting line related to the nettle's action, where it acts either on the underlying tissues or glucose absorption, respectively. This glucose absorption mechanism is based upon enzyme inhibiting detailed (e.g., α-amylase), as shown in **Figure 5**, which is involved in the carbohydrate compounds digestion via the enzymatic pathway.

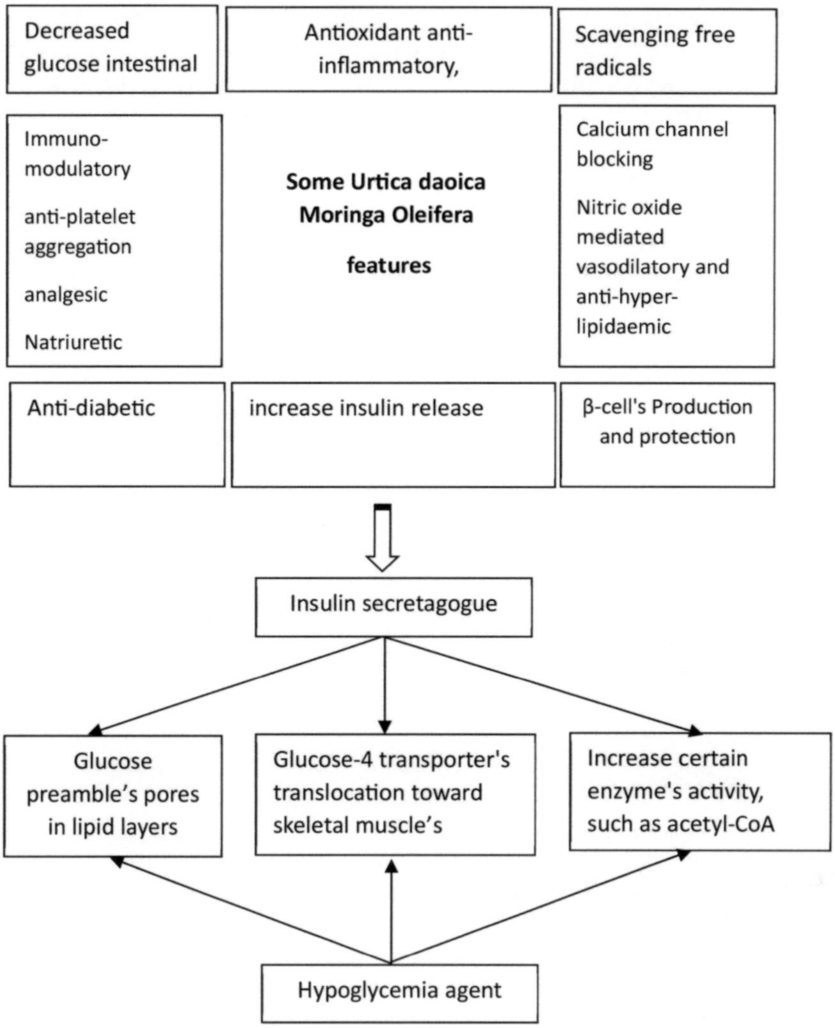

Figure 5.
Both of Urtica dioica and Moringa oleifera properties with main PAM's actions upon human antidiabetic mechanism: Anti-diabetic agents often work by increasing insulin release from the pancreatic β-cells, which are responsible for insulin production. In addition, some compounds have protective effects on β-cells, shielding them from damage and promoting their regeneration. This dual action not only helps regulate blood sugar levels but also preserves the functionality and integrity of pancreatic β-cells, thus contributing to the long-term management of diabetes. Insulin secretagogues increase insulin release from pancreatic β-cells, leading to a reduction in blood glucose levels. They also facilitate glucose transport into cells, improve glucose utilization by skeletal muscle, and increase enzymatic activity for energy production. This overall action helps manage diabetes by improving glycemic control and metabolic function.

4. Conclusion

Both *Moringa oleifera* and *Urtica dioica* present hypoglycaemic properties, giving them the ability to prevent diabetes's onset and even help treat it, owing to their bioactive phytochemicals. Their ability to improve insulin sensitivity, regulate blood glucose levels, mitigate oxidative stress, and reduce inflammation makes them valuable in addressing insulin resistance and related metabolic disorders. Further research and exploration of the mechanisms underlying their effects on diabetes are warranted to harness their full therapeutic potential. The biochemical properties of *Moringa oleifera* and *Urtica dioica* offer valuable insights into their potential as natural remedies for diabetes prevention and treatment. Their diverse range of bioactive compounds and their impact on insulin resistance and glucose metabolism make them promising candidates for further investigation in the field of diabetes management. Nevertheless, understanding the mechanisms of glucose metabolism and homeostasis is crucial for effectively managing diabetes, and these plant models offer valuable insights into this research area. Moreover, studies are needed to explore the specific mechanisms by which *Moringa oleifera* and *Urtica dioica* regulate blood sugar levels.

Author details

Hanane Moummou[1*], Jamal Karoumi[1], Mounir Tilaoui[2], Es-Said Sabir[1], Imane Meftah[3], Mounia Achoch[1], Hicham Chatoui[4], Omar El Hiba[5] and Lahoucine Bahi[6]

1 Private University of Marrakesh, Morocco

2 Sidi Mohamed Ben Abdellah University, Fes, Morocco

3 Sultan Moulay Slimane University, Beni Mellal, Morocco

4 Nursing Training Institute of Marrakesh, Morocco

5 Chouaib Doukkali University, El Jadida, Morocco

6 Royal Institute for Executive Training, Sale, Morocco

*Address all correspondence to: hanane.moummou@gmail.com

References

[1] Kregiel D, Pawlikowska E, Antolak H. *Urtica* spp.: Ordinary plants with extraordinary properties. Molecules. 2018;**23**(7):1664

[2] Mendanha DM, Ferreira HD, Felício LP, Silva EM, Pereira DG, Nunes WB, et al. Modulatory effect of *Byrsonima verbascifolia* (Malpighiaceae) against damage induced by doxorubicin in somatic cells of *Drosophila melanogaster*. Genetics and Molecular Research. 2010;**9**(1):69-77

[3] Leone A, Spada A, Battezzati A, Schiraldi A, Aristil J, Bertoli S. Cultivation, genetic, ethnopharmacology, phytochemistry and pharmacology of *Moringa oleifera* leaves: An overview. International Journal of Molecular Sciences. 2015;**16**(6):12791-12835

[4] Gális I, Onkokesung N, Baldwin IT. New insights into mechanisms regulating differential accumulation of phenylpropanoid-polyamine conjugates (PPCs) in herbivore-attacked *Nicotiana attenuata* plants. Plant Signaling & Behavior. 2010;**5**(5):610-613

[5] Morgan CR, Opio C, Migabo S. Chemical composition of Moringa (*Moringa oleifera*) root powder solution and effects of Moringa root powder on *E. coli* growth in contaminated water. South African Journal of Botany. 2020;**129**:243-248

[6] Mzid M, Ben Khedir S, Bardaa S, Sahnoun Z, Rebai T. Chemical composition, phytochemical constituents, antioxidant and anti-inflammatory activities of *Urtica urens* L. leaves. Archives of Physiology and Biochemistry. 2017;**123**(2):93-104

[7] Yunuskhodzhaeva NA, Abdullabekova VN, Ibragimova KS, Mezhlumyan LG. Amino-acid composition of *Urtica dioica* leaves and *Polygonum hydropiper* and *P. aviculare* herbs. Chemistry of Natural Compounds. 2014;**50**:970-971

[8] Pareek A, Pant M, Gupta MM, Kashania P, Ratan Y, Jain V, et al. *Moringa oleifera*: An updated comprehensive review of its pharmacological activities, ethnomedicinal, phytopharmaceutical formulation, clinical, phytochemical, and toxicological aspects. International Journal of Molecular Sciences. 2023;**24**(3):2098

[9] Ahmed AA, Zain U, Abdulaziz MAO, Riaz U, Iqbal H, Shabir A, et al. Evaluation of the chemical composition and element analysis of *Urtica dioca*. African Journal of Pharmacy and Pharmacology. 2012;**6**(21):1555-1558

[10] Sharifi-Rad J, Quispe C, Herrera-Bravo J, Martorell M, Sharopov F, Tumer TB, et al. A pharmacological perspective on plant-derived bioactive molecules for epilepsy. Neurochemical Research. 2021;**46**(9):2205-2225

[11] Taheri Y, Quispe C, Herrera-Bravo J, Sharifi-Rad J, Ezzat SM, Merghany RM, et al. *Urtica dioica*-derived phytochemicals for pharmacological and therapeutic applications. Evidence-Based Complementary and Alternative Medicine. 2022;**2022**:4024331

[12] Dhouibi R, Affes H, Salem MB, Hammami S, Sahnoun Z, Zeghal KM, et al. Screening of pharmacological uses of *Urtica dioica* and others benefits. Progress in Biophysics and Molecular Biology. 2020;**150**:67-77

[13] Gharsallah K, Rezig L, Msaada K, Chalh A, Soltani T. Chemical composition

and profile characterization of *Moringa oleifera* seed oil. South African Journal of Botany. 2021;**137**:475-482

[14] Wass JA, Stewart PM, editors. Oxford Textbook of Endocrinology and Diabetes. USA: Oxford University Press; 2011

[15] Pfeifer MA, Halter JB, Porte D Jr. Insulin secretion in diabetes mellitus. The American Journal of Medicine. 1981;**70**(3):579-588

[16] Dardari D. Impact de la normalisation rapide de l'hyperglycémie chronique dans la physiopathologie de la neuroarthopathie de Charcot chez les patients vivant avec un diabète [doctoral dissertation]. France: Université Paris-Saclay; 2021

[17] World Health Organization. Definition and Diagnosis of Diabetes Mellitus and Intermediate Hyperglycaemia: Report of a WHO/IDF Consultation. Geneva, Switzerland: WHO Document Production Services; 2006

[18] Cheng YJ, Gregg EW, Geiss LS, Imperatore G, Williams DE, Zhang X, et al. Association of A1C and fasting plasma glucose levels with diabetic retinopathy prevalence in the US population: Implications for diabetes diagnostic thresholds. Diabetes Care. 2009;**32**(11):2027-2032

[19] Bansal N. Prediabetes diagnosis and treatment: A review. World Journal of Diabetes. 2015;**6**(2):296

[20] Goyal A, Gupta Y, Singla R, Kalra S, Tandon N. American diabetes association "standards of medical care—2020 for gestational diabetes mellitus": A critical appraisal. Diabetes Therapy. 2020;**11**:1639-1644

[21] Riddell MC, Sigal RJ. Physical activity, exercise and diabetes. Canadian Journal of Diabetes. 2013;**37**(6):359-360

[22] Mukonzo JK, Namuwenge PM, Okure G, Mwesige B, Namusisi OK, Mukanga D. Over-the-counter suboptimal dispensing of antibiotics in Uganda. Journal of Multidisciplinary Healthcare. 2013;**6**:303-310

[23] Skyler JS. Diabetic complications: The importance of glucose control. Endocrinology and Metabolism Clinics. 1996;**25**(2):243-254

[24] Röder PV, Wu B, Liu Y, Han W. Pancreatic regulation of glucose homeostasis. Experimental & Molecular Medicine. 2016;**48**(3):e219-e219

[25] Reusch JE. Current concepts in insulin resistance, type 2 diabetes mellius, and the metabolic syndrome. The American Journal of Cardiology. 2002;**90**(5):19-26

[26] Hong Z, Xie J, Hu H, Bai Y, Hu X, Li T, et al. Hypoglycemic effect of *Moringa oleifera* leaf extract and its mechanism prediction based on network pharmacology. Journal of Future Foods. 2023;**3**(4):383-391

[27] Amelia D, Santoso B, Purwanto B, Miftahussurur M, Joewono HT. Effects of *Moringa oleifera* on insulin levels and folliculogenesis in polycystic ovary syndrome model with insulin resistance. Immunology, Endocrine & Metabolic Agents in Medicinal Chemistry (Formerly Current Medicinal Chemistry-Immunology, Endocrine and Metabolic Agents). 2018;**18**(1):22-30

[28] Divi SM, Bellamkonda RAMESH, Dasireddy SK. Evaluation of antidiabetic and antihyperlipedemic potential of aqueous extract of *Moringa oleifera* in fructose fed insulin resistant and STZ induced diabetic wistar rats: A comparative study. Asian Journal of Pharmaceutical and Clinical Research. 2012;**5**(1):67-72

[29] Fan S, Raychaudhuri S, Kraus O, Shahinozzaman M, Lofti L, Obanda DN. *Urtica dioica* whole vegetable as a functional food targeting fat accumulation and insulin resistance—A preliminary study in a mouse pre-diabetic model. Nutrients. 2020;**12**(4):1059

[30] Xie J, Qian YY, Yang Y, Peng LJ, Mao JY, Yang MR, et al. Isothiocyanate from *Moringa oleifera* seeds inhibits the growth and migration of renal cancer cells by regulating the PTP1B-dependent src/ras/raf/ERK signaling pathway. Frontiers in Cell and Developmental Biology. 2022;**9**:790618

[31] Siahaan SCP, Santoso B, Widjiati. Effectiveness of *Moringa oleifera* leaves on TNF-α expression, insulin levels, glucose levels and follicle count in *Rattus norvegicus* PCOS model. Diabetes, Metabolic Syndrome and Obesity: Targets and Therapy. 2022;**15**:3255-3270

[32] Huang Z, Wang W, Huang L, Guo L, Chen C. Suppression of insulin secretion in the treatment of obesity: A systematic review and meta-analysis. Obesity. 2020;**28**(11):2098-2106

[33] Sha ZJ, Li CF, Tang SH, Yang HJ, Zhang Y, Li ZY, et al. Efficacy and mechanism of new resource medicinal materia *Moringa oleifera* leaves against hyperlipidemia. Zhongguo Zhong yao za zhi = Zhongguo Zhongyao Zazhi = China Journal of Chinese Materia Medica. 2021;**46**(14):3465-3477

[34] Gu F, Tao L, Chen R, Zhang J, Wu X, Yang M, et al. Ultrasonic-cellulase synergistic extraction of crude polysaccharides from *Moringa oleifera* leaves and alleviation of insulin resistance in HepG2 cells. International Journal of Molecular Sciences. 2022;**23**(20):12405

[35] Afifah SZ, Widianto SKA, Ariesta I. *Moringa oleifera*, Lam. Extract as therapy for insulin resistance through increasing insulin and GLUT-2 expression in pancreatic islet cells of metabolic syndrome rats model. Metabolism - Clinical and Experimental. 2022;**128**:155039. DOI: 10.1016/j.metabol.2021.155039

[36] Mishra K, Talapatra SN. Prediction of toxicity, pharmacokinetics of selected phytochemicals of leaf of drumstick (*Moringa* Sp.) and molecular docking studies on two receptors as insulin tyrosine kinase for antidiabetic potential. Journal of Advanced Scientific Research. 2022;**13**(02):67-75

[37] Alhabeeb M, Gomaa H. The protective effect of *Moringa olifera* against complications of type2 diabetes mellitus in male albino rats.: Effect of *Moringa oleifera* on diabetes. Journal of Qassim University for Science. 2023;**2**(1):1-6

[38] Satrianawaty LD, Christela F, Josua AA, Prabowo S. Pengaruh Ekstrak Daun dan Buah Ketapang Terhadap Malondialdehida Pankreas *Rattus norvegicus* Jantan dengan Hiperglikemia yang Diinduksi Aloksan dan Pakan Tinggi Lemak. Hang Tuah Medical Journal. 2019;**17**(1):66-76

[39] Putri IS, Siwi GN, Budiani DR, Rezkita BE. Protective effect of moringa seed extract on kidney damage in rats fed a high-fat and high-fructose diet. Journal of Taibah University Medical Sciences. 2023;**18**(6):1545

[40] Samakar B, Mehri S, Hosseinzadeh H. A review of the effects of *Urtica dioica* (nettle) in metabolic syndrome. Iranian Journal of Basic Medical Sciences. 2022;**25**(5):543

[41] Ziaei R, Foshati S, Hadi A, Kermani MAH, Ghavami A, Clark CC,

et al. The effect of nettle (*Urtica dioica*) supplementation on the glycemic control of patients with type 2 diabetes mellitus: A systematic review and meta-analysis. Phytotherapy Research. 2020;**34**(2):282-294

[42] Sharma S, Padhi S, Chourasia R, Dey S, Patnaik S, Sahoo D. Phytoconstituents from *Urtica dioica* (stinging nettle) of Sikkim Himalaya and their molecular docking interactions revealed their nutraceutical potential as α-amylase and α-glucosidase inhibitors. Journal of Food Science and Technology. 2023;**60**(10):2649-2658

[43] Shahrokhi M, Koohmanaee S, Haghghi R, Rad AH, Esfandiari MA, Parvinroo S, et al. *Urtica dioica* (nettle) in type 1 diabetes mellitus: A randomized controlled trial. Iranian Journal of Pediatrics. 2023;**33**(5):e137563.

[44] Obanda DN, Ribnicky D, Yu Y, Stephens J, Cefalu WT. An extract of *Urtica dioica* L. mitigates obesity induced insulin resistance in mice skeletal muscle via protein phosphatase 2A (PP2A). Scientific Reports. 2016;**6**(1):22222

[45] Farzami B, Ahmadvand D, Vardasbi S, Majin FJ, Khaghani SH. Induction of insulin secretion by a component of *Urtica dioica* leave extract in perifused Islets of Langerhans and its in vivo effects in normal and streptozotocin diabetic rats. Journal of Ethnopharmacology. 2003;**89**(1):47-53

Chapter 10

Natural Medicine: In-Depth Exploration of *Moringa oleifera*'s Bioactive Compounds and Antimicrobial Effects

Hanane Moummou and Imane Meftah

Abstract

The antimicrobial capabilities of *Moringa oleifera* have garnered significant scientific attention due to its rich array of bioactive compounds. This chapter provides a comprehensive examination of the antimicrobial activities exhibited by various components of the *Moringa oleifera* plant, including seeds, leaves, roots, fruits, and flowers. Notably, Moringa seeds, containing potent 4-(alpha-L-rhamanosyloxy) benzyl isothiocyanates, demonstrate strong antimicrobial effects against a broad spectrum of bacterial strains, including *Bacillus cereus* and *Staphylococcus aureus*, as well as fungi. Furthermore, lectins within Moringa seeds interact with bacterial membranes, impeding growth and viability. Moringa leaves exhibit pronounced antimicrobial actions against both Gram-positive and Gram-negative bacteria, facilitated by phenolic compounds that disrupt essential bacterial functions. Similarly, Moringa roots demonstrate antibacterial and antifungal properties, attributed to compounds like N-benzylethyl thioformate, presenting promising alternatives to conventional antibiotics. Additionally, Moringa fruits and flowers display significant antimicrobial efficacy, with bioactive compounds such as phenols and flavonoids demonstrating activity against common pathogens like *Candida albicans* and *Escherichia coli*. This in-depth analysis underscores the multifaceted antimicrobial potential of *Moringa oleifera*, highlighting pathways for further research and the development of novel antimicrobial agents and nutraceuticals.

Keywords: medicinal plant, *Moringa oleifera*, antimicrobial effect, bioactive compound, microorganism

1. Introduction

The *Moringa oleifera* plant is renowned for its nutritional density and medicinal versatility and is particularly known for its remarkable antimicrobial properties. This chapter delves into the antimicrobial attributes of various components of the *Moringa oleifera* plant, analyzing their mechanisms of action and potential therapeutic applications.

The seeds of *Moringa oleifera* emerge as potent antimicrobial agents, containing 4-(alpha-L-rhamanosyloxy) benzyl isothiocyanates that exhibit striking efficacy

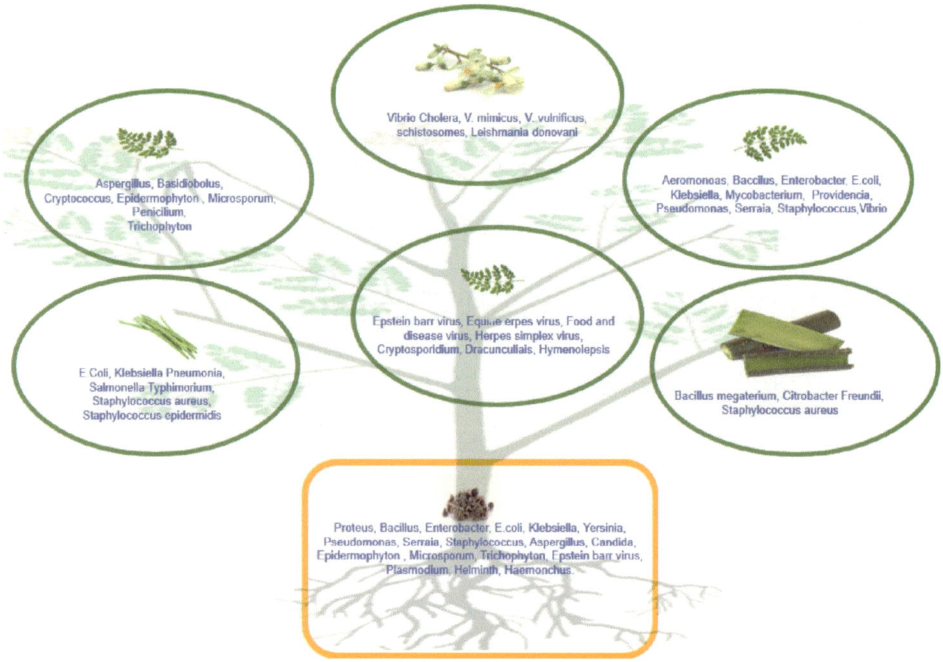

Figure 1.
The antimicrobial activities of various parts of the Moringa oleifera *plant. Specifically, the leaves, seeds, roots, flowers, and pods all exhibit antimicrobial properties. Among these, the leaves stand out for their potent antimicrobial activity against Gram-negative bacteria, with* Escherichia coli *being particularly susceptible. Similarly, the seeds are recognized for their antimicrobial properties. Notably, the roots demonstrate good antibacterial activity against* Escherichia coli, Bacillus subtilis, *and* Staphylococcus aureus, *except for the lateral root. Additionally, the flowers and pods of the plant have been utilized as natural preservatives due to their antimicrobial effects. This comprehensive overview underscores the diverse antimicrobial potential inherent in different parts of the* Moringa oleifera *plan [1].*

against a wide range of bacteria, including *Bacillus cereus* and *Staphylococcus aureus*, as well as certain fungi. Additionally, the presence of lectins in Moringa seeds enhances their antimicrobial effects, as they interact with bacterial membranes, ultimately inhibiting their growth and vitality. Moringa leaves also possess impressive antimicrobial activities, effectively defending against both Gram-positive and Gram-negative bacteria, thanks to the phenolic constituents that disrupt the bacterial mechanism. Similarly, Moringa roots display antibacterial and antifungal compounds, such as the indomitable N-benzylethyl thioformate, offering promising alternatives to conventional antibiotics. Furthermore, Moringa fruits contain bioactive compounds like phenols and flavonoids, which embark on campaigns against well-known microbial adversaries, including *Candida albicans* and *Escherichia coli*. This diverse array of antimicrobial prowess exhibited by *Moringa oleifera* calls for further exploration and innovation in the fields of antimicrobial therapeutics and nutraceuticals, promising to unlock new frontiers in the ongoing pathways against microbial infections (**Figure 1**) [1–3].

2. Antimicrobial seeds activities

Despite the flavonoid coat present in its seeds, Moringa oleifera demonstrates antibiofilm potential against Pseudomonas aeruginosa, Staphylococcus aureus, and

Candida albicans [4] which is discernible through the disc diffusion method [2, 5–7]. Additionally, antimicrobial peptides play a significant role in inhibiting essential enzymes and disrupting cell membranes [8]. Moreover, the Moringa oleifera seeds extract displays antimicrobial activity against Gram-negative bacteria [9, 10] and inhibits bacteriophage replication [11]. Additionally, its antibiotic activity corrects the pathogenic strain actions of *Candida albicans, Staphylococcus aureus*, and *Enterococcus casseliflavus* [12]. Besides, while this extract exhibits weaker effectiveness against *Pseudomonas aeruginosa* and *E. coli* compared to *Bacillus cereus*, it demonstrates strong inhibitory effects against *Bacillus cereus, Staphylococcus aureus*, Mucor species, and Aspergillus species, suggesting potential for treating the related infections caused by these organisms. It also shows inhibitory effects against bacteria such as *Staphylococcus aureus* [13] and Vibrio cholera [12, 14]. The antimicrobial effect of *Moringa oleifera* seeds is primarily attributed to its active components (to moringine, pterygospermine, and 4-(alpha-L-rhamanosyloxy) benzyl isothiocyanates [15]). Besides, two different isothiocyanate compounds exhibit a minimum inhibitory concentration of 1 mg/ml against all tested Gram-positive bacteria and dermatophytic fungi [16].

Lectins, carbohydrate-binding proteins present in Moringa seeds, exhibit diverse biological properties, notably antimicrobial activities. Isolated lectins from *Moringa oleifera* seeds interact with carbohydrates on bacterial membranes, causing damage particularly to species like *Bacillus cereus*, *Bacillus megaterium*, *Micrococcus* sp., *Pseudomonas* sp., *Pseudomonas fluorescens, Pseudomonas stutzeri*, and *Serratia marcescens* [16–18] thereby inhibiting cell growth and cell death (**Figure 2**). Moreover, these lectins and proteins bind specifically to carbohydrate motifs and peptidoglycan components in bacterial cell walls, resulting in membrane damage and disruption of structural integrity. Consequently, there is a leakage of cell contents and activation of apoptotic pathways in bacterial cells, which serves as a defence mechanism against pathogens and inhibits bacterial growth by disrupting essential cellular processes.

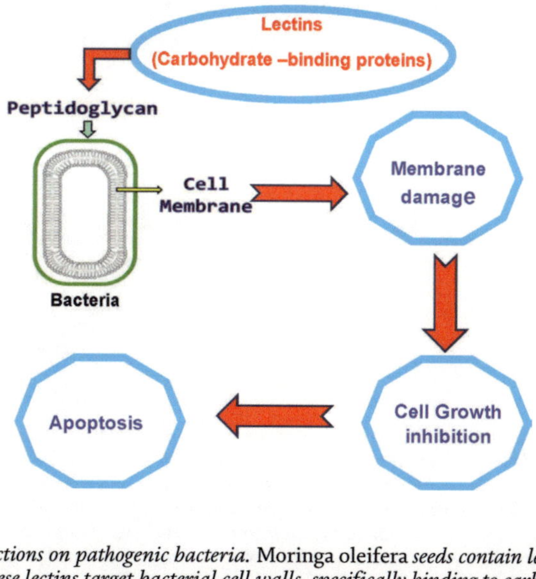

Figure 2.
Lectins SMO pathway's actions on pathogenic bacteria. Moringa oleifera *seeds contain lectins and proteins that bind to carbohydrates. These lectins target bacterial cell walls, specifically binding to carbohydrate motifs and peptidoglycan components. This interaction leads to membrane damage and disrupts the structural integrity of the cell wall, causing leakage of cell contents and activating apoptotic pathways in bacterial cells. This programmed cell death mechanism serves as a defence against pathogens and inhibits bacterial growth by disrupting essential cellular processes.*

3. Antimicrobial leaves activities

Overall, this section highlights the multifaceted antibacterial properties of *Moringa oleifera* leaves, emphasizing their potential as natural antimicrobial agents with diverse mechanisms of action against bacterial pathogens.

Moringa oleifera leaves (MOL) exhibit significant antimicrobial effects against a wide range of bacterial species, including both Gram-positive (e.g., *Staphylococcus aureus*, *Enterococcus faecalis*) and Gram-negative (e.g., *Escherichia coli*, *Pseudomonas aeruginosa*) strains [19, 20]. This antimicrobial action is attributed to the inhibition zones generated by the disc diffusion method, indicative of the effectiveness of MOL against various organisms. The antimicrobial action of Moringa leaves is mediated by

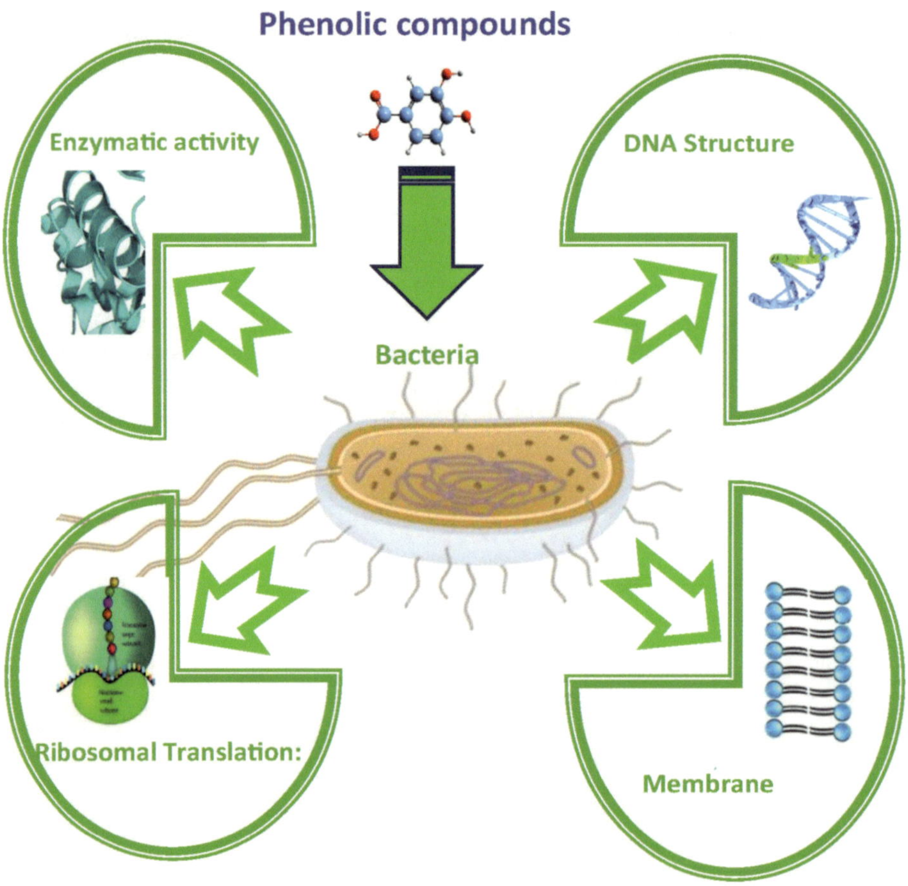

Figure 3.
Main Moringa's phenolic *compounds antibacterial mechanisms* Moringa oleifera *leaves are rich in phenolic compounds, renowned for their antioxidant and antibacterial properties. These compounds play a vital role in the leaves' antibacterial mechanism by impeding bacterial enzymatic activity and interfering with DNA structure upon contact with bacterial cells. By inhibiting key enzymatic processes crucial for bacterial survival and replication, phenolic compounds disrupt vital cellular functions, hindering bacterial proliferation and inducing cellular stress. Moreover, they can directly interact with bacterial DNA, leading to structural alterations that compromise bacterial viability by impeding essential cellular processes like replication and transcription. Additionally, Moringa leaf extracts impact bacterial membranes by interacting with the lipid bilayer, causing destabilization and disruption. This leads to compromised membrane integrity, cell content leakage, and eventual bacterial cell death. Furthermore, interference with ribosomal function by phenolic compounds inhibits protein synthesis and disrupts bacterial translation, further contributing to the antibacterial effect of* Moringa oleifera *leaves.*

phytol, a component derived from chlorophyll that can be transformed into phytanic acid which contributes to the inhibition of bacteria such as *Pseudomonas aeruginosa* and *Staphylococcus aureus* [1]. A necrotrophic plant fungus are also inhibited at 99% within the methanolic leaves extract [2]. Besides, *Moringa oleifera* leaves are rich in phenolic compounds, known for their antioxidant and antibacterial properties. These compounds disrupt bacterial enzymatic activity, interfere with DNA structure, and impact bacterial membranes. Such interactions lead to compromised membrane integrity, cell content leakage, and eventual bacterial cell death. Additionally, plant polyphenols found in Moringa leaves act against bacterial cells through various mechanisms, including interaction with bacterial proteins and cell walls, alteration of membrane permeability, and inhibition of DNA synthesis. The amphipathic nature of polyphenolic compounds plays a significant role in their antibacterial activity (**Figure 3**). Moreover, methanolic extracts of Moringa leaves have shown potential in inhibiting urinary tract infections caused by both Gram-negative and Gram-positive bacteria, including *Klebsiella pneumoniae*, *Escherichia coli*, and *Staphylococcus aureus*.

In DNA, the molecule and hydrophobic core flatness means that polyphenols can penetrate the DNA helix during replication, recombination, and transcription. Moreover, polyphenols can also combine with metals such as CU^{2+} and form complexes that modify DNA stability. In fact, the inhibition mechanism depends on the polyphenol structure and bacterial species. The molecule's favorable hydrophilic or hydrophobic characteristics depend on the action sites. So, the amphipathic phenolic compound action plays a major role in antibacterial activity. Additionally, phenolics also interact with synthetic pathways, such as inhibiting topoisomerase or DNA gyrase activity by polyphenols [21, 22].

4. Antimicrobial roots activities

In this section, the antimicrobial activities of *Moringa oleifera* roots will be investigated, and their potential as a natural remedy against infections will be explored. Thanks to their high content of antimicrobial compounds, such as flavonoids and alkaloids, MO root extracts can inhibit the growth of various harmful bacteria and fungi, including *E. coli* and *Candida albicans*. This famous fight against antibiotic-resistant bacterial strains makes these roots a potential alternative to conventional antibiotics.

Thanks to the presence of compounds, such as flavonoids and phenolic acids, which have been found to disrupt bacterial cell membranes and inhibit enzyme activity. The antimicrobial properties of MO roots make them a promising natural alternative for fighting infections.

Besides, *Moringa oleifera* roots (MOR) are rich in antimicrobial agents and antibacterial activities consequently, and this is due to the powerful antibacterial and fungicidal effects of an active antibiotic known as N-benzylethyl thioformate (an aglycone of deoxyniazimincin). Furthermore, MO's bark (MOB) extract showed strong activity against *Staphylococcus aureus* (most sensitive), *Bacillus megaterium*, *Pseudomonas fluorescens*, and *Citrobacter freundii*. Also, the root bark *Moringa*'s antibacterial and antifungal activities are due to the aglycone of deoxy-niazimicine (N-benzyl, S-ethyl thioformate) [14]. Over and above that, the latter compound is found to be also responsible for these activities in MO root bark. In fact, an effect against *Staphylococcus aureus* was revealed in stem bark [23]. With further research and development, MO roots may be utilized in the future as a safe and effective treatment option for infections [24, 25].

In fact, some studies revealed that none of the elements extracted from *Moringa* roots were of concern for drinking water quality. Extracts from this miraculous plant are used not only in medicine but also in other industries such as water treatment [4].

5. Antimicrobial fruits activities

Research indicates that the bioactive compounds in *Moringa oleifera* fruits offer a range of health benefits, including anti-inflammatory properties and potential therapeutic applications against chronic diseases. The rich array of bioactive compounds underscores the nutritional and medicinal importance of *Moringa oleifera* as a valuable plant for human health and well-being.

The fruit of *Moringa oleifera* (MOF), rich in alkaloids, flavonoids, and steroids, exhibits a notable inhibitory impact on *Candida albicans* cultures, attributed to its steroidal ring structure. This inhibitory effect operates through mechanisms involving protein denaturation and inhibition of spore germination pathways [18]. The complex interaction of bioactive compounds within MOF underscores its potential as a formidable agent against *Candida albicans*, offering new insights into its therapeutic efficacy and prompting further research into its pharmaceutical applications.

The antimicrobial activities of *Moringa oleifera* fruits is an area of research exploring the potential of *Moringa oleifera* fruit extracts to inhibit the growth and activity of microorganisms. These extracts have shown promising antimicrobial properties against a range of bacteria and fungi, including Gram-positive and Gram-negative strains. Studies have identified bioactive compounds in *Moringa oleifera* fruit extracts that contribute to their antimicrobial activity. These compounds include phenols, flavonoids, alkaloids, and glucosinolates. They have been shown to be effective against a range of pathogens, including *Staphylococcus aureus*, *Escherichia coli*, and *Aspergillus niger*. This potential of *Moringa oleifera* fruit as a natural antimicrobial agent suggests its possible use in the development of new antimicrobial drugs or treatments.

6. Antimicrobial flowers activities

Mostly, this part emphasizes the significant therapeutic effects of *Moringa oleifera* flowers, in pharmaceutical and nutraceutical applications owing to their rich array of bioactive compounds. Compounds such as glucomoringin and benzyl glucosinolate are identified as common constituents found in various parts of the Moringa plant, including flowers, stems, pods, leaves, seeds, and roots, which highlights the widespread distribution of bioactive compounds throughout the plant, contributing to its therapeutic versatility.

Additionally, flowers are highlighted as a highly rich source of phenols, flavonoids, and minerals, distinguishing them for their potent antioxidant and antifungal properties [23, 26], which make their nutritional profiles comparable to *Moringa oleifera* leaves, but the creamy color and potentially greater acceptability of flower powder make them more used for food applications [21].

Moreover, emerging research suggests the efficacy of *Moringa oleifera* flowers as a natural remedy for urinary tract ailments, indicating their potential role in improving human health and combating antibiotic resistance [23, 27].

This section underscores also the diverse pharmacological effects of *Moringa oleifera* flowers, including antibacterial, antifungal, anti-inflammatory, and

DOI: http://dx.doi.org/10.5772/intechopen.1005046

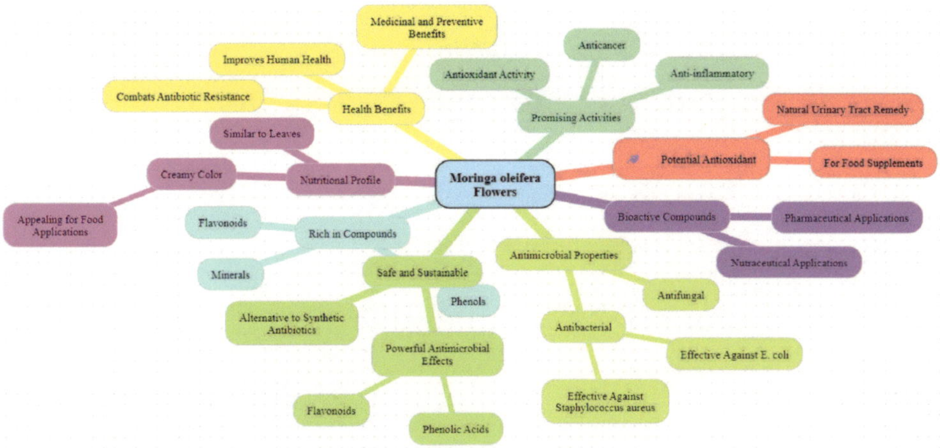

Figure 4.
Moringa oleifera’s *flowers composition, properties and health benefits.*

anticancer properties. Moreover, their antioxidant activity is highlighted, offering a safe and sustainable alternative to synthetic antibiotics.

Figure 4 summarizes the virtues of *Moringa oleifera* flowers.

7. Conclusion and future directions

In summation, the discerning analysis undertaken in this study underscores the promising antimicrobial attributes exhibited by *Moringa oleifera* across a spectrum of fungi. Extracts derived from the seeds, leaves, root bark, fruit, and flowers intricately showcase inhibitory effects on diverse pathogenic strains. The elucidation of specific active components, including 4-(alpha-L-rhamanosyloxy) benzyl isothiocyanates, lectins, phytol, and N-benzylethyl thioformate are paramount in comprehending the complex mechanisms underpinning these antimicrobial actions. This research accentuates the potential of *Moringa oleifera* as a reservoir of natural compounds, offering a fertile ground for the development of antimicrobial agents with tangible applications in the pharmaceutical landscape, thereby contributing substantively to the ongoing global initiatives aimed at combating fungal infections. Further exploration and refinement of these natural compounds stand as imperatives in the trajectory toward effective pharmaceutical solutions.

Moreover, according to previous studies, MO might also be used to prevent antibiotic toxicity. However, further extensive studies should be made to assess the relationship between infections to bring MO compounds to clinical trials as its potential for becoming an antimicrobial drug. Owing to their involvement in nutritional prevented routes, MO is considered as one of the best medicinal plants, providing a tremendous phytochemical effect. According to various studies oscillating from traditional medicine to a bioactive compound, an overview of some bacteria, fungi, and viruses has been listed. In alignment with the previously cited studies, *Moringa*’s full of nutriments and its major key prevention could be confirmed. Furthermore, a better understanding of microbial effects has been established.

Author details

Hanane Moummou[1*] and Imane Meftah[2]

1 Private University of Marrakesh, Morocco

2 Sultan Moulay Slimane University, Beni-Mellal, Morocco

*Address all correspondence to: hanane.moummou@gmail.com

References

[1] Xiao X, Wang J, Meng C, Liang W, Wang T, Zhou B, et al. *Moringa oleifera* Lam and its therapeutic effects in immune disorders. Frontiers in Pharmacology. 2020;**11**:566783

[2] Pareek A, Pant M, Gupta MM, Kashania P, Ratan Y, Jain V, et al. *Moringa oleifera*: An updated comprehensive review of its pharmacological activities, ethnomedicinal, phytopharmaceutical formulation, clinical, phytochemical, and toxicological aspects. International Journal of Molecular Sciences. 2023;**24**(3):2098

[3] Upadhyay P, Yadav MK, Mishra S, Sharma P, Purohit S. *Moringa oleifera*: A review of the medical evidence for its nutritional and pharmacological properties. International Journal of Research and Pharmaceutical Science. 2015;**5**:12-16

[4] Morgan CR. Chemical and antimicrobial properties of *Moringa* (*Moringa oleifera*) root and its impact on water quality [doctoral dissertation]. University of Northern British Columbia; 2020. Available from: https://unbc.arcabc.ca/islandora/object/unbc:59045

[5] Anwar F, Ashraf M, Bhanger MI. Interprovenance variation in the composition of *Moringa oleifera* oilseeds from Pakistan. Journal of the American Oil Chemists' Society. 2005;**82**(1):45-51

[6] Galuppo M, De Nicola GR, Iori R, Dell'Utri P, Bramanti P, Mazzon E. Antibacterial activity of glucomoringin bioactivated with myrosinase against two important pathogens affecting the health of long-term patients in hospitals. Molecules. 2013;**18**(11):14340-14348

[7] Padla EP, Solis LT, Levida RM, Shen CC, Ragasa CY. Antimicrobial isothiocyanates from the seeds of *Moringa oleifera* Lam. Zeitschrift für Naturforschung. Section C. 2012;**67**(11-12):557-564

[8] Suarez M, Entenza JM, Doerries C, Meyer E, Bourquin L, Sutherland J, et al. Expression of a plant-derived peptide harboring water-cleaning and antimicrobial activities. Biotechnology and Bioengineering. 2003;**81**(1):13-20

[9] Anzano A, De Falco B, Ammar M, Ricciardelli A, Grauso L, Sabbah M, et al. Chemical analysis and antimicrobial activity of *Moringa oleifera* Lam. leaves and seeds. Molecules. 2022;**27**:8920

[10] Onsare JG, Arora DS. Antibiofilm potential of flavonoids extracted from *Moringa oleifera* seed coat against *Staphylococcus aureus*, *Pseudomonas aeruginosa* and *Candida albicans*. Journal of Applied Microbiology. 2015;**118**(2):313-325

[11] Al-Jadabi N, Laaouan M, El Hajjaji S, Mabrouki J, Benbouzid M, Dhiba D. The dual performance of *Moringa oleifera* seeds as eco-friendly natural coagulant and as an antimicrobial for wastewater treatment: A review. Sustainability. 2023;**15**(5):4280

[12] Flores B, Ramírez E, Moncada A, Salinas N, Fischer R, Hernández C, et al. Antimicrobial effect of *Moringa oleifera* seed powder against Vibrio cholerae isolated from the rearing water of shrimp (*Penaeus vannamei*) postlarvae. Letters in Applied Microbiology. 2022;**74**(2):238-246

[13] Sun A, Huang Z, He L, Dong W, Tian Y, Huang A, et al. Metabolomic analyses reveal the antibacterial properties of a novel antimicrobial peptide MOp3 from *Moringa oleifera* seeds against *Staphylococcus aureus* and its application in the infecting pasteurized milk. Food Control. 2023;**150**:109779

[14] Mukherjee D, Mukherjee G. Bioprospecting of pods of *Moringa oleifera* Lam. as novel antibacterial agent. Indian Journal of Experimental Biology (IJEB). 2023;**61**(02):131-137

[15] van den Berg J, Kuipers S. The antibacterial action of *Moringa oleifera*: A systematic review. South African Journal of Botany. 2022;**151**:224-233

[16] Chuang PH, Lee CW, Chou JY, Murugan M, Shieh BJ, Chen HM. Anti-fungal activity of crude extracts and essential oil of *Moringa oleifera* Lam. Bioresource Technology. 2007;**98**(1):232-236

[17] Coriolano MC, Brito JS, Ferreira GRS, Moura MC, Melo CML, Soares AKA, et al. Antibacterial lectin from *Moringa oleifera* seeds (WSMoL) has differential action on growth, membrane permeability and protease secretory ability of Gram-positive and Gram-negative pathogens. South African Journal of Botany. 2020;**129**:198-205

[18] Medeiros ML, Alves RR, Napoleão TH, Paiva PM, Coelho LC, Bezerra AC, et al. Anthelmintic effect of a water soluble *Moringa oleifera* lectin in rodents experimentally infected with *Haemonchus contortus*. Parasitology International. 2023;**92**:102656

[19] Ahmed M, Marrez DA, Abdelmoeen NM, Mahmoud EA, Abdel-Shakur Ali M, Decsi K, et al. Proximate analysis of *Moringa oleifera* leaves and the antimicrobial activities of successive leaf ethanolic and aqueous extracts compared with green chemically synthesized Ag-NPs and crude aqueous extract against some pathogens. International Journal of Molecular Sciences. 2023;**24**(4):3529

[20] Almatrafi M. The Effects of Moringa Leaves on Hepatic Lipid Accumulation and Inflammation in a Guinea Pig Model of Hepatic Steatosis. Doctoral Dissertations. 1522. 2017. Available from: https://opencommons.uconn.edu/dissertations/1522

[21] Granella SJ, Bechlin TR, Christ D, Coelho SRM, de Oliveira Paz CH. An approach to recent applications of *Moringa oleifera* in the agricultural and biofuel industries. South African Journal of Botany. 2021;**137**:110-116

[22] Oulahal N, Degraeve P. Phenolic-rich plant extracts with antimicrobial activity: An alternative to food preservatives and biocides? Frontiers in Microbiology. 2022;**12**:753518

[23] Punia J, Singh R. Antioxidant potential and nutritional content of stem, bark and pod of drumstick tree (*Moringa oleifera* Lam.) from semi-arid region of Haryana. Journal of the Indian Chemical Society. 2017;**94**(1):103-110

[24] Kwami WS, Saeed HA, Hamad MNM. Screening the antibacterial activity of *Moringa oleifera* leaves and seeds extract against selected members of bacteria. 2020;**10**(3):121-129

[25] Lobiuc A, Pavăl NE, Mangalagiu II, Gheorghiță R, Teliban GC, Amăriucăi-Mantu D, et al. Future antimicrobials: Natural and functionalized phenolics. Molecules. 2023;**28**(3):1114

[26] Chiș A, Noubissi PA, Pop OL, Mureșan CI, Fokam Tagne MA, Kamgang R, et al. Bioactive compounds in *Moringa oleifera*: Mechanisms of action, focus on their anti-inflammatory properties. Plants. 2023;**13**(1):20

[27] Pop OL, Kerezsi AD, Ciont C. A comprehensive review of *Moringa oleifera* bioactive compounds—Cytotoxicity evaluation and their encapsulation. Food. 2022;**11**(23):3787

Chapter 11

Selenium and Prebiotics as Adjunctive Therapies in Treatment of Graves' Disease

Hanane Moummou, Lahoucine Bahi, Nahid Shamandi, Iman Meftah, Oumnia Akhallaayoune, Mounia Akhallaayoune and Abdelilah El Abbassi

Abstract

Graves' disease (GD), also known as Basedow disease, is an autoimmune disorder leading to excessive production of thyroid hormones (hyperthyroidism). The prevalence of GD varies by region and sex, with the highest onset typically occurring between the ages of 30 and 50. Symptoms include a rapid heart rate, weight loss, heat intolerance, and goiter. Standard treatments involve antithyroid medications, radioactive iodine therapy, or surgery. Multiple studies have linked gut microbiota to the development of thyroid disorders. Recent research has focused on the potential benefits of nutritional interventions, particularly selenium and prebiotics, in managing GD. This chapter aims to provide new insights into the etiology and treatment of Graves' disease through the administration of probiotics and selenium.

Keywords: selenium, prebiotics, Graves' disease, thyroid, adjunctive therapies

1. Introduction

Multiple studies suggest that inadequate blood and tissue levels of specific micronutrients in the nutrient-sufficient range promote and/or sustain autoimmune diseases such as GD [1] and that tumor necrosis factor is a key player in the regulation of microelements [2]. The rare micronutrient deficiency diseases demonstrate the dependence of the thyroid gland on various trace elements [3]; in the economically developed world, however, the widespread availability and the absence of overt deficiency states give little cause for most individuals and their caregivers to pay attention to these potentially pathophysiologic vulnerabilities [4]. Understanding the complex relationships between trace elements and preexisting diseases is crucial for developing targeted therapeutic strategies and improving patient outcomes. Copper and selenium are involved in the initial iodination event as cofactors of the thyroid peroxidase, managing iodine's incorporation into tyrosine residues of thyroglobulin [5].

When GD is treated with thionamide antithyroid drugs (ATD), hypothyroidism develops in a certain percentage of patients after several weeks to months due to the TSH receptor–blocking effect of the thionamide, leading to a decrease in the titer of the newly released antibody [6, 7]. Hypothyroidism might also develop due to the destructive antibody effect on the gland's follicular cells or the occurrence of concomitant Hashimoto's thyroiditis. To alleviate the clinical symptoms of hypothyroidism and to decrease the risk of myxedema myocarditis, treatment is aimed at replacing thyroid hormone [8].

GD is an autoimmune disorder manifested mostly by hyperthyroidism, an increase in the metabolic rate, heat intolerance, weight loss, sweating, fine tremor, insomnia, palpitations, fatigue, goiter, lid lag, and stare due to lid retraction, ophthalmopathy, and dermopathy [9]. Most patients have IgG antibodies against the TSH receptor, stimulation of which leads to gland growth and hormone release. Graves' hyperthyroidism typically fluctuates in severity and often spontaneously resolves, requiring indefinitely suppressive doses of ATD, radioactive iodine treatment, thyroidectomy, or, for carefully selected patients, no definitive therapy [10]. In opposition to the *primum non nocere* principle, a percentage of patients are unable to tolerate methimazole due to intolerance of the drug itself or its minor side effects, including allergic or cholestatic hepatic injury and hematologic toxicity [11]; a percentage choose and adhere to radioiodine therapy due to prior exposure to antithyroid drug side effects, a dislike for their fluctuating symptomatology, social or job-related constraints, or a preference for a single definitive treatment [12].

2. Physiopathology of Graves' disease

Since GD is an autoimmune disease, its onset is usually related to increased intestinal permeability, which is an initiating factor for autoimmune diseases [13]. Increased intestinal permeability combined with an imbalance of beneficial bacteria and dysbiosis, or a subtle impairment of the intestinal immune barrier, might contribute to the onset of autoimmune processes in those who are genetically predisposed [14].

The immune system normally protects the body by patrolling the bloodstream and killing bacteria or viruses, but in individuals who have GD, the immune system produces a type of antibody called thyroid-stimulating immunoglobulin (TSI) [15]. TSI attaches to the surface of thyroid cells, inducing the gland's overactivity. This overactivity of the thyroid leads to the characteristic symptoms of GD, such as an enlarged thyroid, rapid heart rate, nervousness, anxiety, fatigue, weight loss, muscle weakness, and tremors in the hands [9, 14].

The exact cause of GD is unknown, although current research suggests that GD is largely a result of genetic predisposition [16]. It is certainly a multifactorial disease, which involves the interaction between genetic susceptibility and environmental agents such as stress, infections, and certain drugs [14].

2.1 Autoimmune mechanisms

In autoimmune thyroid disease, increased levels of reactive oxygen species are implicated not only in the concept of establishing a proinflammatory effect but also in influencing the differentiation of precursor T-helper and T-regulatory cells into mature cells [17]. Finally, there is a suggestion that selenium is particularly central in influencing the action of the transcription factor TGF beta [18–20], helping to maintain gut barrier integrity and thus enhancing the differentiation of T-regulatory cells and reducing inflammation by decreasing IL-6 and enhancing IL-10 levels [21].

A range of factors from genetics, gender, imbalances in pro- and anti-inflammatory cytokines, and intestinal flora to genetic and environmental factors, such as iodine, selenium, and infectious agents, have been implicated in the etiopathogenesis of Graves' disease [14, 16]. Selenium exerts its antioxidant function by acting as an essential cofactor for the enzyme family glutathione peroxidase and thus reducing the cellular concentration of hydrogen peroxide and organic hydroperoxides, which if they accumulate to mirror levels in tissues, contribute to lipid, DNA, and protein damage, leading to extensive tissue damage and autoimmune conditions [22, 23].

2.2 Role of thyroid-stimulating hormone receptor

The thyroid-stimulating hormone receptor (TSHR) facilitates the action of TSH on the thyroid gland, promoting the growth and proliferation of thyrocytes as well as the production of thyroid hormones [24]. In Graves' disease, thyroid-stimulating autoantibodies mimic TSH, stimulating thyroid cells and causing hyperthyroidism and excessive thyroid hormone production. The binding epitopes for TSHR antibodies on the receptor molecule are well-studied [24–26]. Therefore, the activation of TSH receptor signaling during postnatal development increases the proliferation of benign cells and greatly accelerates the formation of their cancerous offspring [27, 28]. Unlike the current paradigm, mutations of the GNAS1 gene reduce TSHR signaling and, by either inhibiting cAMP production or increasing the Gnαs activity (lack of regulation), slow down the proliferation. Furthermore, in case all three proteins were mutated (TSHR; GNAS1; GNM), TSHR signaling would lose all its meaning if, especially for an embryonic mouse, thyroid-stimulating hormone were necessary. In a recent study, it is alleged that TSHR signaling is preserved during the early stages of thyroid tumorigenesis and that the inability of TSHR-deficient mice to bear an ectopic tumor is unrelated to activation [29].

The thyroid-stimulating hormone (TSH) receptor is a G-protein-coupled receptor that is present in its precursor form during embryonic development and appears on the cell membrane of the thyroid follicular cell on the 19th–21st gestational days in the mouse. At the time of birth, the receptor is present on the surface of the cell and forms a complex mass with other components of the basement membrane [30].

3. Current treatment approaches

3.1 R1: risk factors of Graves' disease; genetic testing for primary (or only) prevention

The 2nd ERA recommended that 11 children born to mothers with Graves' disease, 4 children who have two first-degree relatives with Graves' disease, irrespective of whether it is on the maternal or paternal side, 2 first-degree relatives with Graves' disease (mother and sister), and 3 populations at increased risk of GD based on family history should be tested. However, in the majority, the disease appears unexpectedly [31, 32].

The first question that arises is whom to treat. Since the diagnosis and treatment of Graves' disease are not as straightforward as one might think, many patients are treated without giving them a complete and necessary rundown of the potential risks and benefits of therapy. Additionally, Graves' disease is a unique autoimmune disease, as it is one of the few in which the cause of the autoimmune response is known, as well as the main autoimmune pathogenesis—stimulation of the TSHR by autoantibodies, particularly thyroid-stimulating antibodies (TSAb), and B-lymphocyte hyperactivity. This knowledge has opened the door to numerous therapeutic candidate treatments which interfere with the pathogenesis. Furthermore, treatments of other autoimmune diseases frequently are retrospective observations of benefits or adverse effects of already established treatment strategies. The four Rs discussed herein provide a comprehensive approach for the treatment initiation and monitoring of Graves' disease [33].

3.2 Antithyroid medications

Although the European Thyroid Association recommends consideration of definitive therapy for all patients, some subgroups may benefit from any antithyroid drug therapy, including intolerant patients to thionamides, patients with a large goiter, and young patients who may undergo additional exposure to radiation or surgery during a lifetime [34].

According to the latest American Thyroid Association consensus, long-term low-dose therapy is the recommended dosage plan, with 2–2.5 years of therapy post achieving a euthyroid state serving as the ideal minimum treatment duration. Long-term low-dose therapy is a marriage of withdrawal and short-term low-dose methods, including minimal drug administration with the required length of therapy to achieve a remission effect post achieving a euthyroid state. Long-term low-dose therapy can add 20% of Graves' disease patients who may benefit from improvement in the relapse rate by achieving a prolonged therapy duration [35].

In the treatment of Graves' disease, antithyroid medications can be used as a single therapy or as a bridge to definitive therapy. Four strategies can be employed in the administration of antithyroid medications: block-and-replace, withdrawal, and short-term or long-term low-dose therapy. Treatment with an appropriately low dose has a remission induction effect, while the higher doses influence this action [35].

Controversy remains on the optimal treatment regime for Graves' disease, due to potential side effects with antithyroid medications and relapse after definitive therapy with radioactive iodine or surgery [34, 36]. Although better characterization of patients for the risk of relapse may aid in the decision for definitive therapy, identifying novel adjunctive therapies with this action, such as selenium and prebiotics, is of immense interest [35].

3.3 Radioactive iodine therapy

The use of radioactive iodine (131I) rituximab therapy for GD is often characterized by a rapid onset of hypothyroidism, due to the destruction of the thyroid tissue caused by the radiation emitted by the 131I, which is selectively absorbed by the cells expressing the sodium-iodide symporter. Hypothyroidism is associated with longer remission, higher patient satisfaction, and better overall outcomes, including the prevention of complications related to Graves' disease.

When deciding the optimal therapeutic approach for the patient with newly diagnosed Graves' hyperthyroidism, it is important to bear in mind the possible risks and benefits and present the case in a balanced way, perhaps offering the patient the choice between surgery, antithyroid medication, and radioactive iodine. Before treatment is offered, the patient should ideally be given written information on the aims, side effects, and risks of each treatment option and discuss the preferred options with experienced healthcare professionals (normally an endocrinologist and nuclear medicine physician). It is perfectly reasonable for patients to ask their physician who is not a specialist in the field of Graves' disease of the best course of action to take, such as the GP [37].

3.4 Thyroidectomy

Thyroid carcinoma has an extensive usage of lymph node dissections, which can result in a visible external nerve injury. The patients are subjected to total thyroidectomy with isthmectomy and central neck lymph node dissection. This type of surgery decreases transient hypoparathyroidism, but functional LNT injury is frequently found. The loss of delta mRNA expression ratio (TPO/CDH1) can evaluate the LNT dysfunction compared to the contralateral nerve. The saliva is obtained preoperatively and postoperatively from the operated patients, and it is used to evaluate the delta mRNA expression ratio in the LNT. Synchronous saliva-serum samples are available, offering complementary comparisons for preoperative information on the thyroid gland's malignant state. The saliva-serum comparison from the control group and after a 6-month follow-up indicated that energy metabolism, protein homeostasis, and cellular integrity represent potential biological process pathways.

Thyroidectomy is considered in the case of small or toxic multinodular goiter, in the presence of malignancy, or in the presence of an extensive LNT. The total or subtotal thyroidectomy impacts the LNT regenerating process. The level of mRNA expression of the selenoenzymes decreases progressively from 6 to 12 months post-total thyroidectomy. A scratch wound assay presented that the LNT isolated from patients subjected to total thyroidectomy migrates more slowly compared to cells isolated from healthy patients. Treatment with the concentration of selenium found in the serum of healthy people restored the wound healing ability of the LNT from patients subjected to thyroidectomy. Also, after 24 hours of L-selenomethionine treatment, the level of expressions of mRNA of selenoenzymes GPX1, 2, and 4 was restored [38, 39].

4. Rationale for adjunctive therapies

4.1 Limitations of current treatments

Treatments with iodine and corticosteroids can help control thyrotoxicosis before definitive therapy with antithyroid drugs but do not shorten the average time to remission [40]. Furthermore, all treatments for GD have the risk of side effects and potential drug adverse events, especially hepatic, neuropsychiatric, and hematologic side effects for MMIs and PTUs, and the limited choice in treatment options [41]. RDAs are lacking in the general population and may consequently leave GD patients more vulnerable to a myriad of detrimental effects that mediators released during the inflammatory response can have on the organism [42]. There is a growing interest in the use of supplements for patients with autoimmune disorders to mitigate the release of proinflammatory mediators by modulating oxidative and immune functions.

In vitro and experimental trials with metal-based trace elements like selenium have shown some benefits from lower oxidative stress, reduced circulating proinflammatory cytokines, and increased circulating levels of interleukin 4, an anti-inflammatory cytokine [43]. The ecosystem within and surrounding the digestive tract can also influence the degree of reactivity of the innate and adaptive immune responses occurring in GD. This review aims to highlight the benefits arising from such a diet plan, namely a diet enriched in oligofructose, a prebiotic that can selectively stimulate the activity and growth of beneficial bacteria, acting as a sort of shield against the degree of the immune system's protection from the onslaught of the mediators of the inflammatory response and elicited by an individual's interference [44].

The spectrum of antithyroid drugs and permanent forms of surgical and ablative therapies (complicated with the risks of post-treatment hypothyroidism), currently available for hyperthyroid GD, points out that treatment strategies do not address the innate and adaptive autonomous immune responses that drive the disease [45]. The introduction of treatments that could target the mechanisms of progression of GD may allow earlier treatment efficacy over a long term. Indeed, the main drawbacks of pharmacological treatments with MMI and PTU antithyroid drugs are the lack of efficacy to deliver a lasting remission from the disease and the long time to reach remission [46]. The relentless rate of remission while on medication in antithyroid drugs and the high rate of recurrence of the disease after withdrawal are key factors of medication withdrawal failure [47]. The low remission rate and compliance are even more pronounced in adolescence with a smaller number of patients being in remission, frequent relapse of hyperthyroidism, and difficulties with access to care in this age group [48].

The level of selenium intake has a large contribution to public health [49]. The inadequacy of selenium can lead to a significant decrease in the immune response, which can make the host susceptible to various types of infectious agents [20, 50]. The role of selenium as an immunoregulator has been known for over 30 years and has been shown mainly by increasing the production of proinflammatory cytokines [51]. For decades, the link between thyroid dysfunctions and selenium has been studied [52]. It is known that selenium is the precursor of iodothyronine deiodinases, which determine the synthesis of active hormones. In addition, the antioxidant role of selenoproteins is often emphasized, in particular the antioxidant role in the thyroid. Consequently, the imbalanced intake of selenium plays a significant role in the occurrence of autoimmune thyroiditis and thyroid tumors and development of preconditions for antimicrobial conditions [53]. Thus, the use and dosage of selenium as a therapeutic agent is essential, especially given the different effects on cellular functions such as the endocrine, immune, or other specifically expressed ones [54].

4.2 Potential benefits of selenium and prebiotics

Formerly, selenium was shown to regulate the functioning of the immune system [55]. Since autoimmunity is related to the Th1 type and hyperplasia appears in the thyroid gland, the shift from Th1 to Th2 immune response could help in pathologies related to the immune response [56]. The regulation of the intestinal microflora, IL-10 level increase, and oxidative stress and inflammation suppression are the mechanisms underlying the Se immune modulatory effects [57]. Furthermore, selenium can also increase the level and action of the VIP, which is a potent anti-inflammatory regulator [58]. Thereby, by using prebiotics, it is possible both to alleviate the damage from GD and to build a defense against stimuli provoking the development of autoimmunity [42].

It is well established that a deliberate reduction of oxygen consumption rate is a key strategy of cell defense. Thus, reduction in individual metabolism is a vital role of selenium-containing proteins, such as 15-kDa selenoprotein [59]. In addition to the antioxidant effect, Se supplementation could reduce the inflammatory status [60]. It has been proven that Se has the ability to modulate cytokine profile making it shift from a Th1-mediated (γ-interferon) to a Th2-mediated (IL-10) immune response that is important during autoimmunity [58]. Moreover, it has been shown earlier that selenium-containing copolymers can increase in vitro production of IL-2 [42].

5. Selenium as an adjunctive therapy

Low selenium status (< 80 μg/L) is associated with increased risk of thyroid disease. Increased selenium intake may reduce the risk in areas of low selenium intake [61]. No significant correlation was found between serum selenium levels and the clinical activity and severity of GO, with the exception of the finding that lower serum selenium concentrations were associated with eyelid retraction [62]. It can be assumed that there is a specific concentration of selenium below which complications are likely to appear in patients with GD, particularly those predisposed to immune hypersensitivity due to lifelong selenium deficiency [43]. It is also likely that the use of selenium is recommended to maintain or restore the concentration of selenium in the THM above the critical concentration [63].

At the Institute of Endocrinology and Metabolism in Kiev, Ukraine, 104 patients with GD, aged between 42 and 45 years, were examined for the level of selenium in the serum, the median urinary iodine excretion, relationship between selenium and ioduria levels [64]. The study results show that the concentration of selenium in whole blood testing is a reliable prognostic criterion for the outcome of GD. Selenium supplementation could visibly reduce the serum levels of FT3, FT4, and TPOAb in patients with AITD, but no observable effects were detected on the levels of TSH and TGAb [65]. Decreased plasma selenium levels < 64.32 μg/L, and increased concentrations of Th2 chemokines (e.g., CCL2) < 190 pg/L, may reflect GO disease activity, shedding light on the diagnosis and evaluation of active GO [66].

In several studies, selenium has been shown to reduce oxidative stress in patients with GD. It also can reduce the concentration of antithyroid antibodies, and prevent or mitigate the appearance of its physical symptoms, or the progression of autoimmune thyroiditis [67]. Data on the toxic effects of increased selenium are not the same in vivo and in vitro. High plasma selenium levels are associated with a common cause of death [40]. With that, the clinical course of autoimmune thyroiditis and smoking is not recommended as a source of selenium [68].

Presently, there are not many factors that could change the progression of GD. Those used have undesirable side effects. The search for new preventive or adjunctive agents for the treatment of patients with GD is relevant. The thyroid gland contains a significant amount of selenium, and its effect on thyroid gland function is of interest in autoimmune thyroid [69]. Currently, the role of selenium as a therapy, which reduces inflammatory activity, can slow autoimmune aggression in GD, and may prevent associated diseases, such as heart disease, malignant neoplasms, and movements and maintain fertility, is the subject of research [70].

The main cause of the progression of autoimmune aggression in GD is an increase in its own antigenic stimulation. Factors that could prevent the progression of autoimmune aggression in GD have been studied. Some of them showed their effectiveness in reducing the symptoms of GD. The role of selenium and prebiotics aimed at normalizing the intestinal microflora in the treatment of GD is considered in this review [52].

Graves' disease (GD) is an autoimmune disorder of the thyroid gland characterized by the overproduction of thyroid hormones, the presence of antithyroid peroxidase and antithyroglobulin antibodies, and typical symptoms [58]. Standard therapy for GD includes the use of thionamides, iodine agents, or corticosteroids, ablative therapy, or surgical thyroidectomy. These methods do not affect the basic pathogenetic processes of the autoimmune aggression against thyrocytes [70]. They are directed against the symptoms of GD.

5.1 Biological functions of selenium

Selenium is a nonmetal that is represented in the Periodic Table of the Elements by the chemical symbol Se [55]. It is an element that is rich in biological and economic significance and is a very important element in nutrition. For over 40 years, its importance in function and health has been understood and has been the focus of medical attention (**Figure 1**). Epidemiologic and laboratory studies support the participation of selenium in preventing infection, cancers, and endocrine, autoimmune, and digestive disorders [60]. Many human diseases are accompanied by low blood and tissue levels of selenium, and increased dietary selenium enhances selenium concentrations throughout the body [58]. Because of its capabilities, selenoproteins either play or are partly involved in more than one customarily glutathione-dependent enzymes [71]. As historically documented, selenium, as a medicinal food, has been applied extensively in China for approximately 1000 years [21].

Selenium's main function in the human body is as a component of the 25 selenoproteins, most of which have a strong antioxidative, anti-inflammatory, and antiviral effect [55]. Several selenoproteins have protective and detoxifying functions linked to excessive oxidative stress, which can damage cells and tissues and initiate an autoimmune response [60]. Selenoproteins play a role in the endoplasmic reticulum and in the regulation of the immune and inflammatory response, which might be of importance under inflammatory and autoimmune states [58]. The polyadenine and selenolate bond within the selenoproteins enable glutathione peroxidases and thioredoxin reductases to lower oxidative stress, and the other selenoproteins participate in redox-signaling pathways or work as molecular chaperones [71].

The selenium could exist in organic or inorganic forms. It is implied in many mechanisms such as immunological ones. Besides, disease such as Basedow or Graves' disease is regulated under the selenium action.

5.2 Studies on selenium supplementation in Graves' disease

The aim of this review is to summarize the data on the effectiveness of supplementation with selenium-iodine-laminina1, selenium, and "Revifort" prebiotic in Graves' disease.

The mechanism of selenium in the treatment of Graves' disease is generally believed to be due to its antioxidant effect [58]. An optimal selenium nutritional status in preventing oxidative damage is suggested by its incorporation into a range of selenoenzymes that function as potent intracellular antioxidants. They convert reactive oxygen species into less toxic forms. Therefore, selenium may inhibit inflammatory damage. However, some studies have suggested that selenomethionine and methyl selenocysteine are immunosuppressive agents [42]. The immunomodulatory

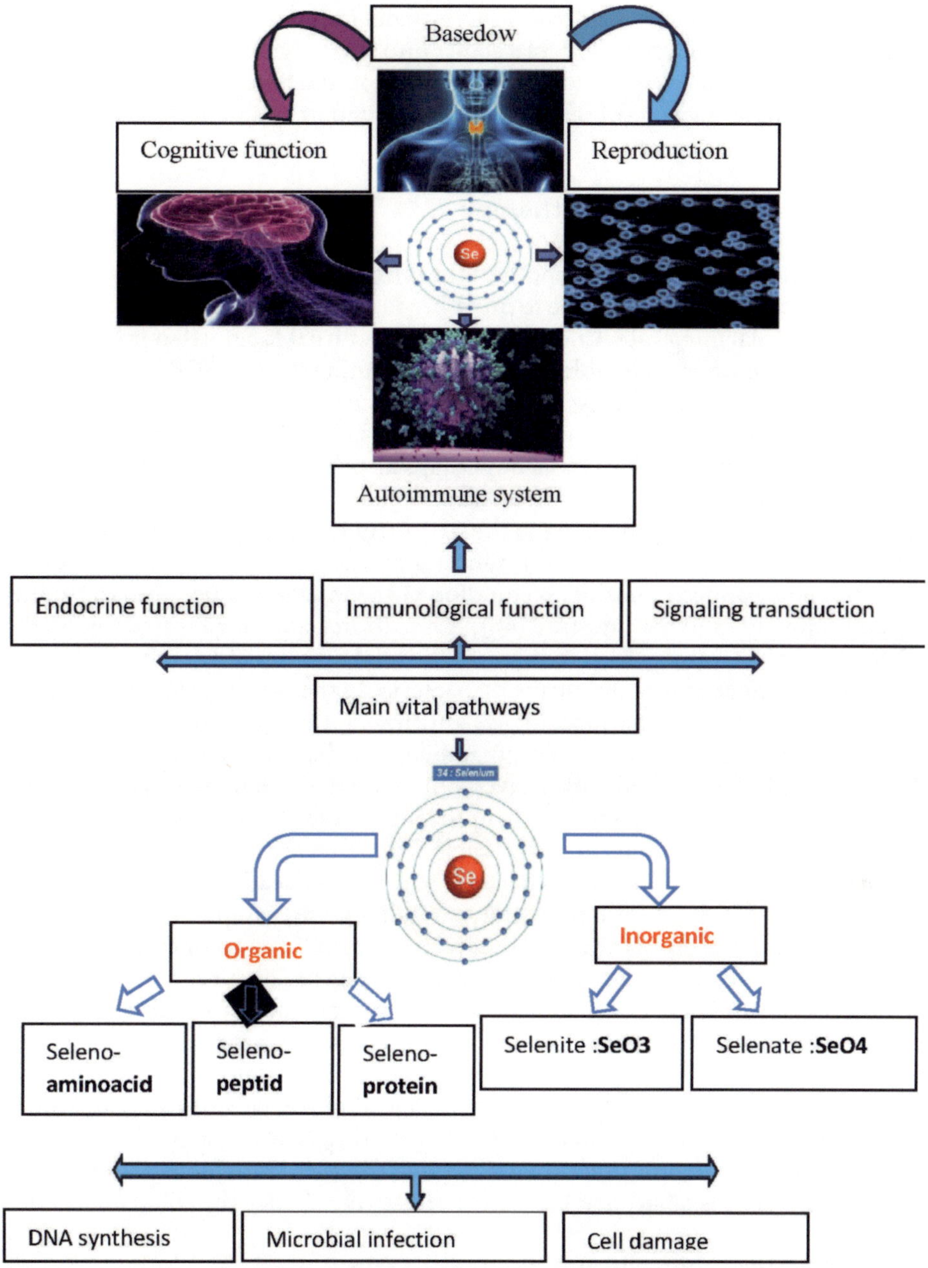

Figure 1.
The selenium implication in vital pathways.

effects of selenium supplementation may be the mechanisms responsible for the treatment of autoimmune thyroid disease [68].

The first study reporting beneficial results of selenium supplementation in Graves' disease was conducted by Contempre et al. in 1991. It used a double-blind, placebo-controlled design in Central Africa. With 50 μg of selenium (as selenomethionine) daily, serum T4 concentrations decreased without a concomitant increase in serum TSH concentrations in the healthy children. Shortly after that, a Polish team reported the beneficial effects of selenium supplementation on oxidative stress by reducing lipid peroxidation. This was done in a randomized, double-blind, placebo-controlled design at a dose of 100 mg per day [72]. These two studies received abundant attention and became the classic papers that promoted the application of selenium supplementation in Graves' disease.

6. Prebiotics as an adjunctive therapy

In autoimmune diseases, the hypothesis of the consumed antibiotics, excess sterilization, and reduced exposure to microbes in modern society is increasing in frequency at an alarming rate. Understanding the external factors that influence these conditions is of considerable interest for obtaining data on SCFA metabolites and improving protection against colitis. On the other hand, prebiotics, designed substrates, were usually fructans directly entering the colon to stimulate microflora to show positive effects [73]. In some or perhaps all other tissues, microflora is an essential factor in the regulation of T cell function. Hence, the more beneficial work in microflora disorders is promising in the treatment of autoimmune diseases, as well as intestinal microbiota [74]. In GD, antibiotics could be applied to treat gut dysbiosis, and the tendency aimed at normal restoration of the interaction between the microbiome, environment, and the intestine [48]. A nutritional additional supplementation has been used as encouragement to increase the total number of Lactobacilli with additional treatment of prebiotic-causing bacteria, in the primary therapy of Graves' disease [75]. Dietary and pharmacological antithyroid therapies, such as methimazole, thiourea derivatives, and potassium iodide, have been used. However, the potential role of probiotics, individually or in combination with prebiotics, has not been sufficiently tested as treatments to either prevent or cure the autoimmune process.

Prebiotics are fermentable, non-digestible fibers that are used to stimulate the growth and/or activity of beneficial bacteria in the colon, leading to improvements in host health [76]. Much interest in prebiotics as adjunctive therapies in the treatment of GD stems from the observation that individuals with thyroid conditions are more likely to have gut dysfunction. Therefore, the idea of using dietary intervention in diseases as a way of mitigating the effects of these diseases is very appealing [73]. Using trivial benign metabolic diseases and non-absorbed dietary products as therapeutic tools seems to be an ideal situation. Their role encompasses detoxification of potential toxin producers, their involvement in nutrient metabolism, substitution, and inhibition of other microflora, or "selective stimulation" [77]. There is a lot of hope in dietary therapy of different functional states and diseases. Supplementation with a non-digestible oligosaccharide is the way to selectively change the colon microflora.

6.1 Role of gut microbiota in autoimmune diseases

The gut mucosal immune system comprises both innate and adaptive immune compartments and is finely regulated by an intricate signaling network [78]. This delicate equilibrium of tolerance and immunity can be perturbed by a variety of exogenous factors, including pathogens, commensal microbiota, drugs, or diet. The onset and progression of gut-related immune-mediated diseases such as asthma, multiple sclerosis, obesity, diabetes, rheumatoid arthritis, depression, and mood disorders are closely related to aberrant changes in the composition or function of the intestinal microbiota [79]. The rapidly increasing global incidence of autoimmune disorders warrants a deeper understanding of the underlying causes, including the environmental factors that may modulate the gut microbiota and, subsequently, the immune system. Up to now, factors contributing to the development of autoimmune diseases have only been partially explained. Initial evidence has highlighted the importance of gut microbiota in disease development and raised the possibility of using bacteria and prebiotic treatments to prevent their onset [74].

The gut microbiota is an integral entity of the human body, both with respect to quantity and diversity, and the microbiome profile is the repertoire of microbial genes present in the microbiota [73]. A highly diverse and stable gut microbiota is a key factor in maintaining good health. Both local (affecting gastrointestinal mucosa) and systemic effects of gut microbiome influence efficient gut functioning and protection [74]. However, possibly the most relevant effect of the gut microbiota on human health is related to the fact that the intestinal microbiota contributes to the regulation of immune homeostasis, maintaining a balanced state of a healthy immune system.

6.2 Evidence for prebiotic use in Graves' disease

A beneficial role for prebiotics, in which some are indigestible oligosaccharides, soluble non-digestible fibers, indigestible sugars, but also anti- and honey drink cutaneous bacteria with the honey-producing lactobacilli and other lactobacilli, is evident by the overall protection offered [78]. Perhaps this explains the transcendent advice of ancient Egyptian texts to drink honey or a mixture of milk and honey to protect the mouth and throat from infection, including inflammation. Both prebiotics, in the form of oligofructose-enriched inulin supplement, and oligofructose act as both pre- and probiotics to decrease the severity of celiac disease, with the former combatting dysbiosis and the latter down-regulating duodenal macrophage activity [74].

The rationale for this intervention lies in the known anti-inflammatory properties of prebiotics, which include the ability to inhibit the growth of unhealthy bacteria such as *Escherichia coli* and the promotion of a beneficial community dwelling of Firmicutes and Bacteroidetes [73, 74]. Specific benefits of prebiotics have been observed in preventing or modifying the manifestations of several autoimmune diseases and Graves' disease, where there is direct evidence for a role for type 1 helper (T-h) and/or other inflammatory cytokines. Enhanced levels of pathogenic bacteria, including *E. coli*, have detrimental effects such as the increased ability of the immune system to promote the deposition of inflammatory and oftentimes pathogenic immunoglobulins in affected organs.

7. Combination therapy

Prospects for the near future: The combination of relatively low-harmful (for the body) doses of SS and several PRTs, which are at the stage of completion of clinical trials, with SS at the treatment stage of GD can provide the highest target therapeutic effect with the minimum harm to the body.

1. It is possible to combine the use of relatively low doses of ATDs with SS and PRTs that can correct the main misconceptions of ATD action [73].

2. It is possible to combine the use of relatively low doses of ATDs with the prescription of therapeutically acceptable amounts of ST without side effects [74].

3. The combined use of organic Se + prebiotics with not exceeding the recommended maximum EC level and increasing the intake of the most favorable ones may

be accompanied by a significantly better management of GD compared to monotherapy. The most important advantage of the proposed hypothesis is not only the achievement of the therapeutic goal in managing GD but also the practically complete absence of side effects from the drugs used, which is very significant.

Hypotheses: According to the scientific data discussed above, we can formulate the following hypotheses.

7.1 Synergistic effects of selenium and prebiotics

Correlation studies showed that certain types of beneficial gut bacteria, particularly a group of bacteria in the Firmicutes phylum, can utilize dietary selenite directly or indirectly and turn toxic selenite into a non-toxic form [78]. Prebiotic compounds cannot be absorbed into the blood because the body does not have the metabolic enzymes to degrade or utilize them. They can be hydrolyzed and degraded in the colon and produce a lot of beneficial metabolites, such as short-chain fatty acids, which provide energy for the epithelium [73, 80]. $The activity of short-chain fatty acids (butyrate) on colonocytes is considered an environmental inducer-regulator of apoptosis and proliferation (**Figure 2**) [81].

Intestinal dysbiosis: leading to impaired gut barrier function and increased intestinal permeability, facilitating antigen entry into circulation and immune system activation. *Antibodies*: in circulation may react with bacterial antigens, enhancing the activation of inflammatory foci within the thyroid. *Short-Chain Fatty Acids (SCFAs)*: The main factor influencing Graves' disease through the gut microbiota, increasing attention is being paid to the immunomodulatory effects of short-chain fatty acids (SCFAs).

Fecal SCFAs technology can be used as a treatment for radiation enteritis in clinical settings (**Figure 3**). Therefore, it is important to explore the interaction of prebiotics and enteritis associated with antithyroid drug treatment. More research on the synergistic effects of selenium and prebiotics is essential.

The supplementation of probiotics with prebiotic fiber elicits a stronger probiotic effect in the treatment of disease [81]. Despite studies supporting the benefits of integrating selenium and prebiotic nutrients into diets, the synergistic effects of these nutrients in the treatment of autoimmune diseases may be due to modulating the

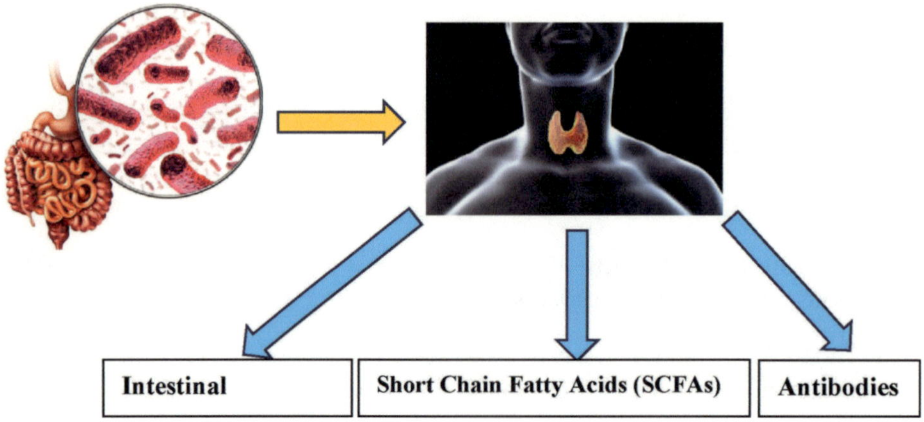

Figure 2.
The impact of microbiota on the thyroid gland.

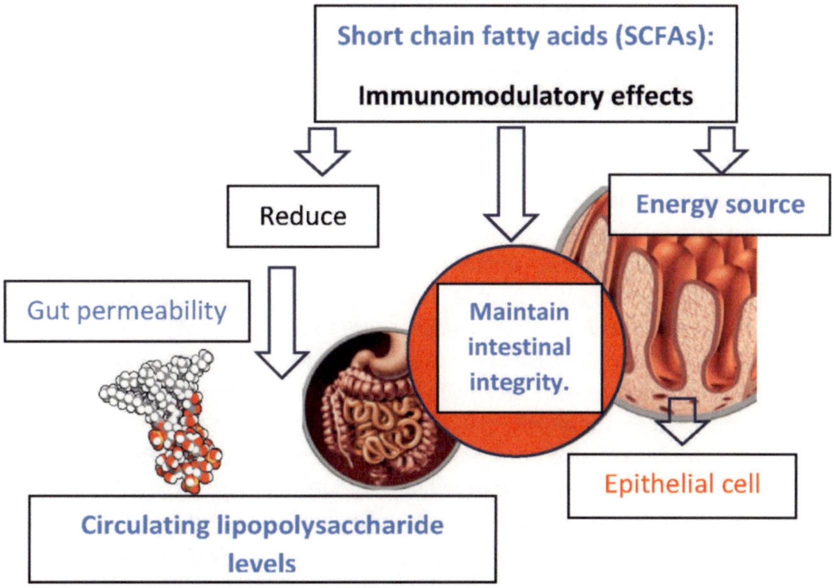

Figure 3.
Short-chain fatty acids (SCFAs) functions.

integrity of the GIT [73]. Selenium has been associated with the increase in the concentration of beneficial bacteria while reducing the inflammatory response. Selenium compounds can improve gut immunity by modulating the gut microbial composition. On the other hand, prebiotics also have the capacity to change the microbiota profile by promoting the proliferation of beneficial bacteria [78]. Although there is limited work on the simultaneous supplementation of selenium yeast and prebiotic fiber in association with the gut, future work might unmask the full potential of this combination.

SCFAs can serve as an energy source for epithelial cells, maintain intestinal barrier integrity, and reduce gut permeability and circulating lipopolysaccharides levels.

8. Safety and adverse effects

Selenium might be effective in reducing thyroid volume in Graves' orbitopathy. While the combination of selenium and probiotics may improve the quality of life in patients with autoimmune thyroiditis. The role of L-selenomethionine in mild Graves hyperthyroidism and the effect of selenium supplementation on antithyroid treatment—results of a prospective, randomized, double-blind, placebo-controlled clinical study. The role of selenium and prebiotics as adjunctive therapies in the treatment of Graves' disease. Adjuvanta: they represent an alternative in the adjuvant treatment of diseases like hyperthyroidism. They are safe medications with a strong anti-inflammatory and protective action of the thyroid. The most common adverse effects are minor allergies for probiotics and gastrointestinal symptoms for selenium [82].

8.1 Potential risks and monitoring

The geographical location of natural habitats of selenium-enriched plants should be kept in mind in the differential diagnosis, including the patient dietary history. In cases of new thyrotoxicosis occurrences treated with selenium monotherapy, the possibility of contamination of selenium-containing tablets with other substances should be considered. Similar signs and symptoms may also occur if the initial loading and maintenance doses are miscalculated or overdosed. In these instances, measuring serum selenium levels is unlikely to expedite the diagnostic process. In countries where a transitory oversupply of selenium has occurred, in vitro fertilized human egg donors may have been exposed and the thyroid of future generations should be monitored [83, 84].

While many patients have had safe treatment using oral selenium as monotherapy at 100–200 mcg per day and long-term intakes from food and supplements of approximately 800 mcg per day are rated as safe, it is important to exclude selenium as a contributing factor to type 2 hyperthyroidism due to ingestion of high dietary selenium levels, for example, from overuse of sports nutrition supplements. A recent meta-analysis suggests that the high level of both selenium content in maternal blood and breast milk is associated with an increased risk of thyroid autoantibodies in neonates and in Graves' disease, which may also bear relevance for Graves' disease generally. Patients with recent onset of symptoms of thyrotoxicosis together with a palpable goiter and characteristic signs of selenium excess, such as garlic breath and a metallic taste, should have the metabolic consequence of any organic selenium determined [85, 86].

9. Future directions

Facilitation of dietary modification for GD is important as the ingestion of Se, through foods or supplements and/or prebiotics as components of healthy diets, is an important adjunctive treatment as discussed in this review. Exploration of the treatment and nutritional complications of comorbid GD found in a large European cohort would provide valuable insights into the practicalities of integrating adjunctive diet and bacterial re-balancing therapies [82]. Tools for the clinical assessment of gastrointestinal health and prompt adjunctive treatments for many patients and their carers would be beneficial. Clinical questions related to the onset differential to insidious and prompt medical therapy and adjunctive therapies in relation to dietary and bacterial precautions warrant further investigation [87].

As discussed in this chapter, innovative approaches to the management of GD which recognize the impact of gastrointestinal microbiota and the importance of nutritional co-factors such as Se are emerging. Research targeting the gut environment and the interaction of the bacteria on optimum functioning of the HPT axis and resultant immune adaptations for thyroid homeostasis support the pursuit of novel, biologically plausible, and cost-effective treatments. To capitalize on the full therapeutic benefits of adjunctive treatment by including Se or prebiotic therapy in the medical management of GD, more well-designed, appropriately powered clinical trials are required. Flow-through research studies that explore the significant clinicogenomic interactions that are so important for Se and gut health need to be identified in GD patients [76, 82].

9.1 Research gaps and opportunities

The concept of co-existence and/or interaction between these two agents, as well as other factors within the GI tract that help in shaping and maintaining the microbiome in disease, is an important theme of current research. Studies done under controlled conditions provide valuable information about the individual effects of the given agent on the microbiome, while early stages of GD are mostly examined in in vitro and animal models. However, real progress is achieved when results obtained in separate studies are put together and new, more advanced hypotheses are drawn. To better understand this complex problem, certain issues regarding the application and usefulness of selenium and prebiotics need to be resolved. It is doubtful whether studies presented so far, based mostly on subjective and state-dependent symptoms and signs of severe GD that have not been identified in the very early stages of GD, may suggest that these agents might have potential benefits in the treatment of the entire spectrum of GD. The determination of the optimal and appropriate duration of selenium supplementation for GD, as well as the proper selection of the most appropriate prebiotic compound and the required Prebiotic Index (PI), which could at best be obtained by matching certain prebiotics with certain probiotic species, optimized in each patient. The implementation of such a program would require the determination and validation of standard molecular and microbiological methods, as well as the extended cost-utility analyses in collaboration with other professionals, including dietitians, microbiologists, and industry [88, 89].

In this review, we described clinical evidence that might suggest the use of selenium and prebiotic fibers as adjunctive therapy during GD as both agents may be of some benefit to patients with GD. However, these effects, observed at a very early disease stage, probably by affecting autoimmunity, may not be so prominent and of substantial advantage in the advanced stages of GD when symptoms are present and first-line therapy might be applicable. Now, both agents are considered as nutritional supplements. However, in our opinion, they should be treated as substances that interact with the gastrointestinal tract environment, which should be taken systematically at the proper time, in the proper dose, by the proper subgroup of patients [90].

10. Conclusion

Prebiotics and dietary fibers can have a unique positive effect on the course of Graves' disease due to the lack of side effects. However, it must be remembered that the flora of the intestine is specific for each person, and expenses can grow quickly. Therefore, the use of fiber polymers from various sources and combinations of several sources (so-called prebiotic combinations) in the prevention and complex therapy of Graves' disease is the goal of further scientific search. A sufficiently profitable method, with the maximum specified therapeutic effect, could be the use of low or medium doses of single strains of probiotics, with the selection of the desired strains, and then a special phase that cannot be avoided: "personalized" to the sensitivity of the strain. At this point, the patient should initially benefit from the participation of a nutritionist, a gastroenterologist, and a laboratory for personalized medicine, cooperating during the preclinical phase of this therapeutic model.

Graves' disease can cause a significant reduction in the quality of life and an increase in the costs of medical care. Conventional therapy using antithyroid drugs, radioactive iodine, and thyroid surgery is not suitable for some patients due to ineligibility, intolerance, or concerns about the side effects of therapy. Currently, the search continues for new methods of comprehensive treatment and means to improve traditional methods known for many years. This chapter proposes a combined treatment that includes the pathogenetic use of microelements, including selenium, Zn, and prebiotics, using drugs and functional food products based on dietary fibers, probiotics, and trace elements. Administering these methods can improve the efficacy of basic therapy aimed at eliminating the thyrotoxicosis syndrome, autoimmune inflammation, and the restoration of euthyroid function.

Author details

Hanane Moummou[1*], Lahoucine Bahi[2], Nahid Shamandi[3], Iman Meftah[4], Oumnia Akhallaayoune[5], Mounia Akhallaayoune[5] and Abdelilah El Abbassi[5]

1 Private University of Marrakech, Morocco

2 Royal Institute for the Training of Youth and Sports Leaders, Moulay Rachid National Sports Center, Salé, Morocco

3 National Health Service, Craigavon, United Kingdom

4 Sultan Moulay Slimane University, Beni Mellal, Morocco

5 University CADI AYYAD of Marrakech, Morocco

*Address all correspondence to: hanane.moummou@gmail.com

References

[1] Song Q, Ji X, Xie Y. Effects of antioxidant supplementation on Graves' disease: A meta-analysis. Journal of Clinical Pharmacy and Therapeutics. 2023;(1):5587361. DOI: 10.1155/2023/5587361

[2] Schmitz H, Fromm M, Bentzel CJ, Scholz P, Detjen K, Mankertz J, et al. Tumor necrosis factor-alpha (TNFα) regulates the epithelial barrier in the human intestinal cell line HT-29/B6. Journal of Cell Science. 1999;**112**(1):137-146. DOI: 10.1242/jcs.112.1.137

[3] Wróblewski M, Wróblewska J, Nuszkiewicz J, Pawłowska M, Wesołowski R, Woźniak A. The role of selected trace elements in oxidoreductive homeostasis in patients with thyroid diseases. International Journal of Molecular Sciences. 2023;**24**(5):4840. DOI: 10.3390/ijms24054840

[4] Ritchie H, Roser M. Micronutrient Deficiency: Who is Most Affected by the "Hidden Hunger" of Micronutrient Deficiency? Our World in Data; England and Wales; 2017. Available from: https://ourworldindata.org/micronutrient-deficiency

[5] Kim MJ, Kim SC, Chung S, Kim S, Yoon JW, Park YJ. Exploring the role of copper and selenium in the maintenance of normal thyroid function among healthy Koreans. Journal of Trace Elements in Medicine and Biology. 2020;**61**:126558. DOI: 10.1016/j.jtemb.2020.126558

[6] Azizi F, Abdi H, Amouzegar A, Habibi Moeini AS. Long-term thionamide antithyroid treatment of Graves' disease. Best Practice & Research Clinical Endocrinology and Metabolism. 2023;**37**(2):101631. DOI: 10.1016/j.beem.2022.101631

[7] Liu L, Lu H, Liu Y, Liu C, Xun C. Predicting relapse of Graves' disease following treatment with antithyroid drugs. Experimental and Therapeutic Medicine. 2016;**11**(4):1453-1458. DOI: 10.3892/etm.2016.3058

[8] Al-Mansour M, Maglan AF, Altayeb MK, Faraj LA, Felimban EA, Aga SS, et al. The risk of developing lymphoma among autoimmune thyroid disorder patients: A cross-section study. Disease Markers. 2022;**2022**:1-8. DOI: 10.1155/2022/4354595

[9] Pokhrel B, Bhusal K. Graves Disease. [Updated 2023 Jun 20]. In: StatPearls [Internet]. Treasure Island (FL): StatPearls Publishing; Jan 2024. Available from: https://www.ncbi.nlm.nih.gov/books/NBK448195/

[10] Genovese BM, Noureldine SI, Gleeson EM, Tufano RP, Kandil E. What is the best definitive treatment for Graves' disease? A systematic review of the existing literature. Annals of Surgical Oncology. 2013;**20**(2):660-667. DOI: 10.1245/s10434-012-2606-x

[11] Karmisholt J, Andersen SL, Bulow-Pedersen I, et al. Long-term methimazole therapy in graves' hyperthyroidism and adverse reactions: A Danish multicenter study. European Thyroid Journal. 2022;**11**(3):e220031. DOI: 10.1530/ETJ-22-0031

[12] Campennì A, Avram AM, Verburg FA, Iakovou I, Hänscheid H, de Keizer B, et al. The EANM guideline on radioiodine therapy of benign thyroid disease. European Journal of Nuclear Medicine and Molecular Imaging. 2023;**50**(11):3324-3348. DOI: 10.1007/s00259-023-06274-5

[13] Ilchmann-Diounou H, Menard S. Psychological stress, intestinal barrier dysfunctions, and autoimmune disorders: An overview. Frontiers in Immunology. 2020;**11**. DOI: 10.3389/fimmu.2020.01823

[14] Antonelli A, Ferrari SM, Ragusa F, Elia G, Paparo SR, Ruffilli I, et al. Graves' disease: Epidemiology, genetic and environmental risk factors and viruses. Best Practice & Research Clinical Endocrinology and Metabolism. 2020;**34**(1):101387. DOI: 10.1016/j.beem.2020.101387

[15] Dumont JE, Maenhaut C, Christophe D, Roger PP. Thyroid regulatory factors. In: Endocrinology: Adult and Pediatric. Philadelphia, USA: Elsevier; 2016. pp. 1297-1321.e8. DOI: 10.1016/B978-0-323-18907-1.00075-5

[16] Ploski R, Szymanski K, Bednarczuk T. The genetic basis of graves disease. Current Genomics. 2011;**12**(8):542-563. DOI: 10.2174/138920211798120772

[17] Yarosz EL, Chang C-H. The role of reactive oxygen species in regulating T cell-mediated immunity and disease. Immune Network. 2018;**18**(1). DOI: 10.4110/in.2018.18.e14

[18] Kryczyk-Kozioł J, Prochownik E, Błażewska-Gruszczyk A, Słowiaczek M, Sun Q, Schomburg L, et al. Assessment of the effect of selenium supplementation on production of selected cytokines in women with Hashimoto's thyroiditis. Nutrients. 2022;**14**(14):2869. DOI: 10.3390/nu14142869

[19] Kieliszek M, Bano I, Zare H. A Comprehensive Review on Selenium and Its Effects on Human Health and Distribution in Middle Eastern Countries. Biological Trace Element Research; 2022:**200**(3):971-987. DOI: 10.1007/s12011-021-02716-z

[20] Arthur JR, Nicol F, Beckett GJ. The role of selenium in thyroid hormone metabolism and effects of selenium deficiency on thyroid hormone and iodine metabolism. Biological Trace Element Research. Sep 1992;**34**(3):321-325. DOI: 10.1007/BF02783686. PMID: 1384621

[21] Zhang X, Zhang L, Xia K, Dai J, Huang J, Wang Y, et al. Effects of dietary selenium on immune function of spleen in mice. Journal of Functional Foods. 2022;**89**:104914. DOI: 10.1016/j.jff.2021.104914

[22] Sun Y, Wang Z, Gong P, Yao W, Ba Q, Wang H. Review on the health-promoting effect of adequate selenium status. Frontiers in Nutrition. 2023;**10**. DOI: 10.3389/fnut.2023.1136458

[23] Zoidis E, Seremelis I, Kontopoulos N, Danezis G. Selenium-dependent antioxidant enzymes: Actions and properties of selenoproteins. Antioxidants. 2018;**7**(5):66. DOI: 10.3390/antiox7050066

[24] Holthoff H-P, Uhland K, Laszlo Kovacs G, Reimann A, Adler K, Wenhart C, et al. Thyroid-stimulating hormone receptor (TSHR) fusion proteins in Graves' disease. Journal of Endocrinology. 2020;**246**(2):135-147. DOI: 10.1530/JOE-20-0061

[25] Chistiakov DA. Thyroid-stimulating hormone receptor and its role in Graves' disease. Molecular Genetics and Metabolism. 2003;**80**(4):377-388. DOI: 10.1016/j.ymgme.2003.09.001

[26] Smith TJ. TSHR as a therapeutic target in Graves' disease. Expert Opinion on Therapeutic Targets. 2017;**21**(4):427-432. DOI: 10.1080/14728222.2017.1288215

[27] Chu YD, Yeh CT. The molecular function and clinical role of thyroid stimulating hormone receptor in

cancer cells. Cells. 2020;**9**(7):1730. DOI: 10.3390/cells9071730

[28] Larsen CC, Karaviti LP, Seghers V, Weiss RE, Refetoff S, Dumitrescu AM. A new family with an activating mutation (G431S) in the TSH receptor gene: A phenotype discussion and review of the literature. International Journal of Pediatric Endocrinology. 2014;**2014**:1-6. DOI: 10.1186/1687-9856-2014-23

[29] Zhang H, Kong Q, Wang J, Jiang Y, Hua H. Complex roles of cAMP–PKA–CREB signaling in cancer. Experimental Hematology and Oncology. 2020;**9**:1-13. DOI: 10.1186/s40164-020-00191-1

[30] De Felice M, Di Lauro R. Thyroid development and its disorders: Genetics and molecular mechanisms. Endocrine Reviews. 2020;**41**(5):738-765. DOI: 10.1210/er.2003-0028

[31] Mooij CF, Cheetham TD, Verburg FA, Eckstein A, Pearce SH, Léger J, et al. European Thyroid Association Guideline for the management of pediatric Graves' disease. European Thyroid Journal. 2022;**11**(1):e210073. DOI: 10.1530/ETJ-21-0073

[32] Xie H, Chen D, Zhang J, Yang R, Gu W, Wang X. Characteristics of Graves' disease in children and adolescents in Nanjing: A retrospective investigation study. Frontiers in Public Health. 2022;**10**:993733. DOI: 10.3389/fpubh.2022.993733

[33] Dong H, Gong M, Guo Y, Xia Q. New therapeutic horizon of graves' hyperthyroidism: Treatment regimens based on immunology and ingredients from traditional Chinese medicine. Frontiers in Pharmacology. 2022. DOI: 10.3389/fphar.2022.862831

[34] Kahaly GJ, Bartalena L, Hegedüs L, Leenhardt L, Poppe K, Pearce SH. 2018 European thyroid association guideline for the management of graves' hyperthyroidism. European Thyroid Journal. 2018;**7**(4):167-186. DOI: 10.1159/000490384

[35] Ross DS, Burch HB, Cooper DS, Greenlee MC, Laurberg P, Maia AL, et al. 2022 American thyroid association guidelines for diagnosis and management of hyperthyroidism and other causes of thyrotoxicosis. Thyroid. 2022;**32**(2):354-371. DOI: 10.1089/thy.2021.0105

[36] Villagelin D, Romaldini JH, Santos RB. Outcomes in relapsed Graves' disease patients following radioiodine or prolonged low dose of methimazole treatment. Thyroid. 2015;**25**(12):1285-1292. DOI: 10.1089/thy.2015.0231

[37] Perros P, Basu A, Boelaert K, et al. Postradioiodine Graves' management: The PRAGMA study. Clinical Endocrinology (Oxf). 2022;**97**: 664-675. DOI: 10.1111/cen.14719

[38] Pattou F et al. Impact of lymph node dissection on postoperative complications of Total thyroidectomy in patients with thyroid carcinoma. Cancers. 2022;**14**(21):5462. DOI: 10.3390/cancers14215462

[39] Back K, Lee J, Cho A, Choe JH, Kim JH, Oh YL, et al. Is total thyroidectomy with bilateral central neck dissection the only surgery for papillary thyroid carcinoma patients with clinically involved central nodes? BMC Surgery. 29 Jun 2022;**22**(1):251. DOI: 10.1186/s12893-022-01699-5

[40] De Almeida R, McCalmon S, Cabandugama PK. Clinical Review and Update on the Management of Thyroid Storm. Missouri Medicine. 2022;**119**(4):366-371

[41] Taylor PN, Vaidya B. Side effects of anti-thyroid drugs and their

impact on the choice of treatment for thyrotoxicosis in pregnancy. European Thyroid Journal. 2012;**1**(3):176-185. DOI: 10.1159/000342920

[42] Garbo S, Di Giacomo S, Łażewska D, Honkisz-Orzechowska E, Di Sotto A, Fioravanti R, et al. Selenium-Containing Agents Acting on Cancer—A New Hope? Pharmaceutics. 2023;**15**(1):104. DOI: 10.3390/pharmaceutics15010104

[43] Sahebari M, Rezaieyazdi Z, Khodashahi M. Selenium and Autoimmune Diseases: A Review Article. Current Rheumatology Reviews. 2019;**15**(2):123-134. DOI: 10.2174/1573397114666181016112342

[44] Liu Y, Tang S, Feng Y, et al. Alteration in gut microbiota is associated with immune imbalance in Graves' disease. Frontiers in Cellular and Infection Microbiology. **14**:1349397. DOI: 10.3389/fcimb.2024.1349397

[45] Clark AR. Morshed SA, Latif R, Davies TF. Delineating the autoimmune mechanisms in Graves' disease. Immunology Research. 2012;**54**(1-3):191-203. DOI: 10.1007/s12026-012-8312-8

[46] Butt MI, Riazuddin M, Joueidi F, Waheed N. Antithyroid Drugs in the Management of Graves' Disease: A Friend and Foe. Cureus. 2023;**15**(3):e36028. DOI: 10.7759/cureus.36028

[47] Léger J, Carel JC. Hyperthyroidism in childhood: Causes, when and how to treat. Journal of Clinical Research in Pediatric Endocrinology. 2013;**5**:50-56. DOI: 10.4274/jcrpe.854

[48] Lee ACH, Kahaly GJ. Novel Approaches for Immunosuppression in Graves' Hyperthyroidism and Associated Orbitopathy. European Thyroid Journal. 2020;**9**:17-30. DOI: 10.1159/000508789

[49] Wu Y, Yu Z. Association between dietary selenium intake and the prevalence of hypertension: Results from the National Health and Nutrition Examination Survey 2003-2018. Frontiers in Immunology. 2024;**15**:1338745. DOI: 10.3389/fimmu.2024.1338745

[50] Avery JC, Hoffmann PR. Selenium, Selenoproteins, and Immunity. Nutrients. 2018;**10**(9):1203. DOI: 10.3390/nu10091203

[51] Huang Z, Rose AH, Hoffmann PR. The role of selenium in inflammation and immunity: From molecular mechanisms to therapeutic opportunities. Antioxidants & Redox Signaling. 2012;**16**(7):705-743. DOI: 10.1089/ars.2011.4145

[52] Knezevic J, Starchl C, Tmava Berisha A, Amrein K. Thyroid-Gut-Axis: How Does the Microbiota Influence Thyroid Function?. Nutrients. 2020;**12**(6):1769. DOI: 10.3390/nu12061769

[53] Larsen CB, Winther KH, Cramon PK et al. Selenium supplementation and placebo are equally effective in improving quality of life in patients with hypothyroidism. European Thyroid Journal. 2024;**13**(1):e230175. DOI: 10.1530/ETJ-23-0175

[54] Varlamova EG, Turovsky EA, Blinova EV. Therapeutic Potential and Main Methods of Obtaining Selenium Nanoparticles. International Journal of Molecular Sciences. 2021;**22**(19):10808. DOI: 10.3390/ijms221910808

[55] Filippini T, Fairweather-Tait S, Vinceti M. Selenium and immune function: A systematic review and meta-analysis of experimental human studies. The American Journal of Clinical Nutrition. 2023;**117**(1):93-110. DOI: 10.1016/j.ajcnut.2022.11.007

[56] Lee YC. Synergistic effect of various regulatory factors in TH1/TH2 balance; immunotherapeutic approaches in asthma. International Journal of Biomedical Science. 2008;**4**(1):8-13

[57] Fan Y, Xu S, Zhang H, et al. Selenium supplementation for autoimmune thyroiditis: A systematic review and meta-analysis. International Journal of Endocrinology. 2014;**2014**:904573. DOI: 10.1155/2014/904573

[58] Ramos-Leví AM, Marazuela M. Pathogenesis of thyroid autoimmune disease: The role of cellular mechanisms. Endocrinología y Nutrición. 2016;**63**(8):421-429. DOI: 10.1016/j.endoen.2016.09.005

[59] Ye R, Huang J, Wang Z, Chen Y, Dong Y. The Role and Mechanism of Essential Selenoproteins for Homeostasis. Antioxidants (Basel). 2022;**11**(5):973. DOI: 10.3390/antiox11050973

[60] Gholizadeh M, Khalili, A, Roodi PB, et al. Selenium supplementation decreases CRP and IL-6 and increases TNF-alpha: A systematic review and meta-analysis of randomized controlled trials. Journal of Trace Elements in Medicine and Biology. 2023;**79**:127199. DOI: 10.1016/j.jtemb.2023.127199

[61] Wu Q, Rayman MP, Lv H, et al. Low population selenium status is associated with increased prevalence of thyroid disease. The Journal of Clinical Endocrinology & Metabolism. 2015;**100**(11):4037-4047. DOI: 10.1210/jc.2015-2222

[62] Kim TH, Ko J, Kim BR, Shin DY, Lee EJ, Yoon JS. Serum Selenium Levels in Patients with Graves Disease: Associations with Clinical Activity and Severity in a Retrospective Case-control Study. Korean Journal of Ophthalmology. 2022;**36**(1):36-43. DOI: 10.3341/kjo.2021.0146

[63] Wang YS, Liang SS, Ren JJ et al. The Effects of Selenium Supplementation in the Treatment of Autoimmune Thyroiditis: An Overview of Systematic Reviews. Nutrients. 2023;**15**(14):3194. DOI: 10.3390/nu15143194

[64] Kravchenko VI, Grossman AB, Rakov O, et al. Selenium supply and thyroid condition in Grave's disease in the region of iodine deficiency. Problems of Endocrine Pathology. 2021;**75**(1):26-33

[65] Zuo Y, Li Y, Gu X, Lei Z. The correlation between selenium levels and autoimmune thyroid disease: A systematic review and meta-analysis. Annals of Palliative Medicine. 2021;**10**(4):4398408-4394408. DOI: 10.21037/apm-21-449

[66] He M, Wang Y, Wang J, et al. The potential markers involved in newly diagnosed graves' disease and the development of active graves' orbitopathy. Cytokine. 2020;**127**:154998. DOI: 10.1016/j.cyto.2020.154998

[67] Song, Q, Ji X., Xie, Y. Effects of Antioxidant Supplementation on Graves' Disease: A Meta-Analysis. Journal of Clinical Pharmacy and Therapeutics. **2023**(1):5587361. DOI: 10.1155/2023/5587361

[68] Duntas LH. Selenium and the thyroid: A close-knit connection. The Journal of Clinical Endocrinology & Metabolism. 2010;**95**(12):5180-5188. DOI: 10.1210/jc.2010-0191

[69] Contempre B, Dumont JE, Ngo B, Thilly CH, Diplock AT, Vanderpas J. Effect of selenium supplementation in hypothyroid subjects of an iodine and selenium deficient area: The possible danger of indiscriminate

supplementation of iodine-deficient subjects with selenium. The Journal of Clinical Endocrinology and Metabolism. 1991;**73**(1):213-215. DOI: 10.1210/jcem-73-1-213

[70] He Q, Dong H, Gong M, et al. New Therapeutic Horizon of Graves' Hyperthyroidism: Treatment Regimens Based on Immunology and Ingredients From Traditional Chinese Medicine. Frontiers in Pharmacology. 2022;**13**:862831. DOI: 10.3389/fphar.2022.862831

[71] Sturniolo G, Mesa J. Selenium supplementation and autoimmune thyroid diseases. Endocrinología y Nutrición. 2013;**60**(8):423-426

[72] Zheng H, Wei J, Wang L, et al. Effects of Selenium Supplementation on Graves' Disease: A Systematic Review and Meta-Analysis. Evidence-Based Complementary and Alternative Medicine. 2018;**2018**:3763565. DOI: 10.1155/2018/3763565

[73] Afzaal M, Saeed F, Shah YA, et al. Human gut microbiota in health and disease: Unveiling the relationship. Frontiers in Microbiology. 2022;**13**:999001. DOI: 10.3389/fmicb.2022.999001

[74] Sadeghpour Heravi F. Gut Microbiota and Autoimmune Diseases: Mechanisms, Treatment, Challenges, and Future Recommendations. Current Clinical Microbiology Reports. 2024;**11**(1):18-33. DOI: 10.1007/s40588-023-00213-6

[75] Ji J, Jin W, Liu SJ, Jiao Z, et al. Probiotics, prebiotics, and postbiotics in health and disease. MedComm. 2023;**4**(6):e420. DOI: 10.1002/mco2.420

[76] Shu Q, Kang C, Li J, et al. Effect of probiotics or prebiotics on thyroid function: A meta-analysis of eight randomized controlled trials. PLoS ONE. 2024;**19**(1):e0296733. DOI: 10.1371/journal.pone.0296733

[77] Zhou P, Chen C, Patil S, Dong S. Unveiling the therapeutic symphony of probiotics, prebiotics, and postbiotics in gut-immune harmony. Frontiers in Nutrition. 2024;**11**:1355542. DOI: 10.3389/fnut.2024.1355542

[78] Wang X, Yuan W, Yang C, et al. Emerging role of gut microbiota in autoimmune diseases. Frontiers in Immunology. 2024;**15**:1365554. DOI: 10.3389/fimmu.2024.1365554

[79] Xu H, Liu M, Cao J, et al. The Dynamic Interplay between the Gut Microbiota and Autoimmune Diseases. Journal of Immunology Research. 2019;**2019**:7546047. DOI: 10.1155/2019/7546047

[80] Giri PS, Shah F, Dwivedi MK. Probiotics and prebiotics in the suppression of autoimmune diseases. In Probiotics in the prevention and management of human diseases. Academic Press; 2022. pp. 161-186. DOI: 10.1016/B978-0-12-823733-5.00019-2

[81] Liu XF, Shao JH, Liao YT, et al. Regulation of short-chain fatty acids in the immune system. Frontiers in Immunology. 2023;**14**:1186892. DOI: 10.3389/fimmu.2023.1186892

[82] Kahaly GJ, Riedl M, König J, et al. Double-blind, placebo-controlled, randomized trial of selenium in graves hyperthyroidism. The Journal of Clinical Endocrinology & Metabolism. 2017;**102**(11):4333-4341. DOI: 10.1210/jc.2017-01736

[83] Liu L, Wang L, Tong L, Wang F, Fan B. A review of plant selenium-enriched proteins/peptides: Extraction,

detection, bioavailability, and effects of processing. Molecules. 2023;**28**(3):1223. DOI: 10.3390/molecules28031223

[84] Wang J, Hu L. Selenium-enriched plant foods: Selenium accumulation, speciation, and health functionality. Frontiers in Plant Science. 2023. Available from: https://www.frontiersin.org/articles/10.3389/fpls.2023.1001223/full

[85] Ventura M, Melo M, Carrilho F. Selenium and Thyroid Disease: From Pathophysiology to Treatment. International Journal of Endocrinology. 2017;**2017**:1297658. DOI: 10.1155/2017/1297658

[86] Schomburg L, Riese C, Michaelis M, et al. Synthesis and metabolism of thyroid hormones is preferentially maintained in selenium-deficient transgenic mice. Endocrinology. 2006;**147**(3):1306-1313. DOI: 10.1210/en.2005-1089

[87] Chung CW, Jung KY, Jung EH, et al. Efficacy of selenium supplementation for mild-to-moderate Graves' ophthalmopathy in a selenium-sufficient area (SeGOSS trial): Study protocol for a phase III, multicenter, open-label, randomized, controlled intervention trial. Trials. 2023;**24**(1):272. DOI: 10.1186/s13063-023-07282-4

[88] Maftei NM, Raileanu CR, Balta AA, et al. The potential impact of probiotics on human health: An update on their health-promoting properties. Microorganisms. 2024;**12**(2):234. DOI: 10.3390/microorganisms12020234

[89] Whelan K. Mechanisms and effectiveness of prebiotics in modifying the gastrointestinal microbiota for the management of digestive disorders. The Proceeding of the Nutrition Society. 2013;**72**(3):288-298. DOI: 10.1017/S0029665113001262

[90] Bilal JM, Wong HC, Jayaweera J. Refractory Graves' disease dramatically responded to adjunctive colestyramine: Case report and literature review. European Congress of Endocrinology. 2022;**81**:EP1213. DOI: 10.1530/endoabs.81.EP1213